The Body in Motion

Other books by Theodore Dimon, Jr.

The Elements of Skill:
A Conscious Approach to Learning

The Undivided Self:
Alexander Technique and the Control of Stress

Anatomy of the Moving Body, **Second Edition:**
A Basic Course in Bones, Muscles, and Joints

Your Body, Your Voice:
The Key to Natural Singing and Speaking

The Body in Motion

Its Evolution and Design

Theodore Dimon, Jr., EdD

Illustrated by G. David Brown

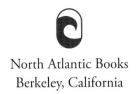

North Atlantic Books
Berkeley, California

Published by
North Atlantic Books
P.O. Box 12327
Berkeley, California 94712

Cover art © iStockphoto.com/Comotion Design
Cover design by Brad Greene
Book design by G. David Brown
Illustrations by G. David Brown
Printed in the United States of America

The Body in Motion: Its Evolution and Design is sponsored by the Society for the Study of Native Arts and Sciences, a nonprofit educational corporation whose goals are to develop an educational and cross-cultural perspective linking various scientific, social, and artistic fields; to nurture a holistic view of arts, sciences, humanities, and healing; and to publish and distribute literature on the relationship of mind, body, and nature.

North Atlantic Books' publications are available through most bookstores. For further information, visit our website at www.northatlanticbooks.com or call 800-733-3000.

Library of Congress Cataloging-in-Publication Data

Dimon, Theodore.
  The body in motion : its evolution and design / Theodore Dimon Jr.
       p. ; cm.
   ISBN 978-1-55643-970-4
1. Musculoskeletal system—Anatomy. 2. Musculoskeletal system—Evolution.
3. Human locomotion. 4. Human locomotion. I. Title.
   [DNLM: 1. Musculoskeletal System—anatomy & histology. 2. Biomechanics.
3. Movement. 4. Musculoskeletal Physiological Phenomena. WE 101 D582b 2010]
   QM100.D563 2010
   611'.7—dc22

                                                                      2010021590

3 4 5 6 7 8 9 UNITED 16 15 14 13 12

To Walter Carrington, with gratitude and appreciation

Contents

Illustrations

11. The Suspensory Muscles of the Throat

12. The Spiral Musculature

13. The Miracle of the Human Form

Preface

The Body in Motion: Its Evolution and Design is based on a series of lectures presented at the Dimon Institute from 1996–2005. Its purpose is to provide a comprehensive look at our wonderful and unique anatomical design. An earlier series of lectures, published as *Anatomy of the Moving Body* (North Atlantic Books, 2001), provided a basic introduction to musculoskeletal anatomy—a working vocabulary of the muscles, bones, and joints that make up the human body. *The Body in Motion* delves more deeply into the subject of how these pieces function as a working whole.

This book is written for students and professionals interested in human movement—educators, bodywork practitioners, physical therapists, medical clinicians, actors, dancers, and anyone interested in understanding anatomy from the perspective of how we're designed to move and function.

There are a number of people who have helped, directly and indirectly, in the making of this book. First I would like to thank Seymour Simmons, my friend and colleague, for his constant support and advice, and for generously allowing me to use his drawing of the Winged Victory of Samothrace at the end of the book.

I would like to thank Dena Davis for her early reading of the manuscript; Richard Grossinger and North Atlantic Books; Jessica Sevey, editor at North Atlantic Books; Brad Green for his cover design: and Judy Gitenstein, editor and publishing consultant, for her advice and support.

Thanks to Anne Everly, Lab Manager in the Herpetology Department at Harvard University, for helping with technical questions on comparative anatomy.

Thanks to Dan Marcus, my friend and colleague, for his excellent editing of the manuscript.

I would like to thank G. David Brown for his book design and superb illustrations. I am lucky to have found such a wonderful collaborator for this and future projects.

Finally, I would like to express my gratitude to Walter Carrington, my teacher and mentor, whose depth of knowledge of functional anatomy forms the foundation for much of what I have learned and written about on this subject.

Introduction

Among the impressive array of machines which humans have invented, there is none that even remotely compares to the subtle and marvelous complexity of the human body. Our capacity for skilled movement, our upright posture, our hands, vision, and the other senses—all are marvels of engineering and design. But why do we possess this design, and how did we become this way? At first glance, many of the seemingly arbitrary details of our anatomy—the bony protrusions of the shoulder girdle, the spine, our intricate musculature—seem to defy full understanding. Yet each of these structures, when examined in terms of its functional design, proves to be uniquely suited for its particular purpose. This book will examine our anatomical design and make sense of the complex structures of the human body in the context of the specific functions they serve.

The topic of our anatomical design, as will become clear in the following pages, falls into two categories. The first deals with specific bodily systems such as the hand and shoulder girdle. Perhaps because so much of what we know about the shoulder girdle and hand is derived from dissections of the human body and detailed studies of its movement, anatomy books—even ones that specialize in movement—tend to focus on technical and quantitative descriptions of muscles, bones, and joints that are often obscure and difficult to understand. Because the subject seems inherently technical, it seems that unless we learn all these details, we'll never really understand how the different parts of the body work.

But such technical descriptions do not do justice to the reality of how these remarkable structures actually work. In simple terms, the shoulder girdle is basically a shallow socket that supports the levers of the upper arm. Because the arms in humans have become adapted for manipulation, this socket is highly movable so that the arm can have as broad a range of motion as possible. Once we understand this, many of the features of the shoulder girdle, such as the shape of the scapula, the function of the clavicle, and the movements we can make at the shoulder, become easy to understand. The hand is also quite complex, but when we look in simple terms at how it works and how the thumb is designed to oppose the fingers, many of the details we thought were important become unnecessary, and the entire thing makes sense in a way we didn't think possible. In this book, we'll look at the various systems in the body and, by understanding what they do in common sense terms, make sense of their anatomical design and their specific parts.

Another factor which tends to complicate the subject of anatomy is the use of language. Because it is based on scientific and technical terminology, anatomy seems to represent a specialized body of knowledge available only to those who have been initiated into this subject by virtue of their scientific background. But most anatomical terms are simply descriptive names given by the Romans and Greeks to parts of the body they needed to identify. When we get behind this language, we demystify the subject and see muscles, bones, and joints for what they are: parts of a complex machine that do things and make sense in the context of what they do. In the following pages, we'll avoid technical language as much as possible, looking instead at how things work and then naming the various parts afterward.

The second theme of this book focuses on our overall design. Exercise and bodywork systems often speak in general terms about muscle groups that need strengthening, larger muscle systems and lines of force, and different ways of training or releasing muscles—all giving the impression of a general framework for how the body works. But most of these systems have been developed by dancers, trainers, or massage therapists who are trying to train the body to look better or get stronger by strengthening or releasing muscle groups; they are not based on a real knowledge or study of how the musculoskeletal system is actually designed to work as a total system in activity. The human body is capable of an amazing array of activities. We can walk on two feet and perform a vast repertoire of movements; by coordinating dozens of muscles throughout the body, we create and form the sounds of speech; using our finely controlled and sensitive hands, we're able to master skills of incredible subtlety and complexity. Yet none of these actions would be possible if we had not evolved our distinctively human upright posture. In order for us to be able to use our hands or control our voices with the required precision, evolution had to work out an elegant upright support system that enables us to perform specific actions and skills—when it works as it's designed to work—with effortless efficiency.

This larger upright system is the basic system on which all the other systems—such as breathing and voice—depend. We can perform breathing exercises to make specific improvements, but unless we understand the total design on which breathing is based, we are working at a huge disadvantage, since this larger design is the single most important factor influencing breathing. The same is true of the health and functioning of specific muscle groups such as the lower back. Various methods promise to elongate, strengthen, and release the back muscles by employing exercises or stretching methods. But the back muscles are inextricably linked with our upright posture, and the only way these muscles can function properly is in the context of this larger system. Even awareness exercises, which tend to make us feel more relaxed and balanced because they are more holistic in approach, cannot be effective if they are not based on a positive concept of how the body is designed to work. A true practice of awareness must be based not on movement or relaxation but on a genuine understanding of how the musculoskeletal system is actually designed to work in activity.

This is not to say that therapeutic methods or awareness practices are completely invalid. Many situations warrant physical therapy, stretching, and treatment. But such systems can't substitute for a working knowledge of how the body is designed to function as a total system in action. When it comes to musculoskeletal functioning, the most important anatomical knowledge we can possess is an understanding of how the body is designed to operate in action based on its total functional design. In this book, we'll look in detail at how the body works as a total system, understand how specific systems relate to this general system, and examine how the body is designed to work as a coordinated whole based on this larger design.

In an even broader sense, our upright design is not just about movement but is directly linked to our higher faculties. The human body is the most versatile moving machine one can imagine. It is capable of producing a greater range of activities, with greater precision, than that of any animal on the planet. To control all these movements, we have evolved that most sophisticated of organs, the human brain, which manages an enormously complex set of functions with remarkable efficiency. Our highly evolved brain, however, is directly linked to our upright design, without which we could not have developed speech or the use of the hands. The musculoskeletal system is indeed a remarkable moving machine, but viewing muscles and bones in purely mechanical terms hardly begins to do justice to the range and beauty of our anatomical design. It is not an overstatement to say that the human body is the vehicle of the soul, for without it, none of our singular human achievements—not even those that are considered purely intellectual or abstract—would be possible. The hand, for instance, is not simply a system of levers that makes it possible to grasp and manipulate objects, nor is it merely a sensory organ; it is in fact the instrument which makes possible many of our greatest technological and artistic achievements. It allows us to explore our world, to fashion instruments, to touch a loved one, and to create works of art. It is, to put it simply, an extension of the brain, without which the brain as we know it could not have evolved. The muscles that support upright posture, our shoulders, limbs, and voice—all are tangible aspects of our higher selves. To understand our physical design is to understand the underpinnings of our intellectual, social, and artistic lives.

1. The Origins of Movement

One of our most distinctive human attributes—and the one that most concerns those of us who are attempting to make sense of our musculoskeletal design—is movement. Like many other vertebrates, we are capable of moving in very complex and sophisticated ways. Vertebrates move by contracting muscles which are attached to bones. The bones form joints with other bones and therefore act as levers; the muscles are motors which move the levers. Some animals can swim underwater, some can run at high speed, and still others can fly. Because we are balanced up on two feet, we are capable of an unusual range of movements, such as the ability to walk and run, to twist and rotate our bodies, to use our arms and hands in various ways, and to produce speech. But all vertebrates, in one way or another, possess the ability to produce movement by contracting muscles which move bones.

Bones, Muscles, and Movement

When we observe the complexity of the human musculoskeletal design, it is difficult to fathom how bones and muscles originated, and why they are so intricately arranged. But this complex system of bony levers and muscles evolved in a definite way and for definite reasons. If you observe a fish swimming, it is easy to see that it mainly uses its muscles and bones to propel itself through the water by levering its flexible spine and tail from side to side. Apart from action of the fins and jaw, a fish doesn't have any other movement options because it lacks other bones and thus other means of hinging or moving parts of its body (Fig. 1-1).

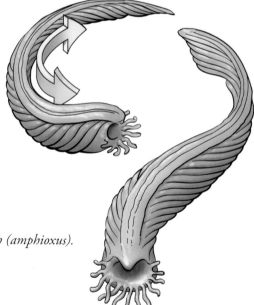

Figure 1-1. A primitive fish (amphioxus).

This simple pattern of movement provides a clue to the origin of vertebrate locomotion. Primitive, one-celled creatures are capable of only the crudest sort of movement; many simply float about aimlessly in their watery environment. As one-celled creatures developed into more complex multicellular animals, some of these developed a long tubular gut for processing food more efficiently, with an opening at one end for taking in the food and at the other for expelling waste. In order to acquire food more efficiently, however, movement through the water in the direction of the food was required. Accordingly, some creatures developed a primitive spine, or notochord—a flexible beam that ran down the length of the body and prevented the body from telescoping when it flexed from side to side—with muscles arranged longitudinally along either side of this central axis. By contracting first one side of the body and then the other, the muscles produced undulating motions which propelled the fish through the water, making it possible to reach food that was otherwise inaccessible (Fig. 1-2).

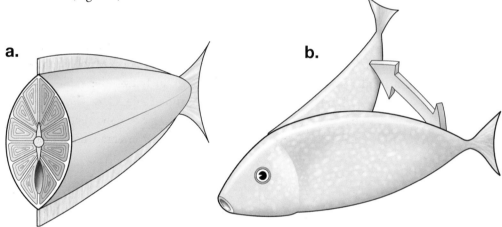

Figure 1-2. Lateral flexion in a fish:
a. muscles on both sides of notochord or spine; b. lateral flexion.

In some species of fish this primitive spine developed into a series of solid vertebrae with protrusions and struts, or ribs, which served as attachments for the muscles. Bone and muscle began to work together in a partnership to produce forward motion through the water. Muscles along the spine became the first motors, and the bony segments of the spine the first levers, for producing vertebrate locomotion through space.

The musculoskeletal system thus originated with the spine and the muscles that acted upon it to create lateral undulating motions that moved the animal through the water. Lateral flexion of the spine, in fact, became the foundation of all vertebrate movement. Thousands of marine animals still move this way, and many amphibians and reptiles, when they move on land, utilize a similar movement to advance their limbs. Even humans, in the earliest stages of life, laterally flex the spine, thus recapitulating this distant stage of their evolutionary heritage.

The Head and Its Central Role in Movement

This evolution of a tubular gut with a mouth at the front end and muscles arranged along the primitive spine was accompanied by several other essential developments. In order to find food, the area around the mouth became specially adapted for perceiving food sources by detecting the presence of molecules in the water (the sense of smell), sensing vibrations caused by the movement of other objects in the water (the sense of hearing), and perceiving images produced by light (vision). As the front end of the evolving fish became more and more sensitive to the presence of food, an increasingly sophisticated cluster of neurons, or brain, was required for processing this information and directing movement. In addition, the mouth developed into a movable jaw which could hinge and thereby capture and seize prey. The front part of the fish, which now housed the jaw, the sensory organs, and the brain, had evolved into a true head—a bony structure articulated with, but distinct from, the rest of the spine.

This "leading segment" of the spine is an essential component of vertebrate design. Muscles along the length of the body move the fish in a forward direction, based on sensory input coming into the front end. In other words, the movement of the body—the action of the lever and motors of spine and muscles—is organized in relation to the head. Thus a head articulated with a bony spine, and a musculature that acts to produce movement in the service of the head, form the blueprint from which all subsequent vertebrate life forms developed.

Four-Footed Animals and the Role of Posture in Movement

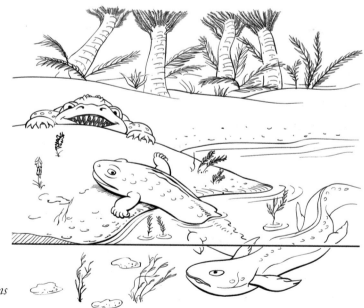

This arrangement further evolved when certain fish developed muscular fins for moving about in shallows, which enabled them to crawl onto land in search of food or to avoid predators (Fig. 1-3). The fins became functional levers, with complex muscular arrangements for acting on these levers, ending

Figure 1-3. Early amphibians coming onto land.

up in terrestrial animals as varied as rodents, dinosaurs, and humans. In this sense, the limbs of rodents, dinosaurs, and humans are nothing more than highly evolved fins.

To use levers on land, however, requires support against gravity. In a marine environment, a fish is buoyed up by the water and therefore lives in a world that is virtually gravity-free. Animals on land, however, have to contend with the pull of gravity; to move efficiently in space, they must first raise themselves off the ground. Some reptiles accomplish this task with their bellies close to the ground and their legs splayed out to the sides; dinosaurs and mammals walked and ran with their legs more directly underneath them, making it possible to move quickly and efficiently on land. Here, the spine comes into play in a completely new way, functioning as a kind of bridge for supporting the body on the forelimbs at one end of the bridge and the hind limbs at the other.

The musculature of terrestrial animals thus serves a dual function: first, it produces overt movement by acting upon bones as levers; second, it counteracts the tendency of these levers to buckle so that, as the animal moves about, the body can be supported on its four limbs. The overt function of muscles in producing movement now takes places against the background of muscular tone, which serves to maintain the supporting limbs in a stable postural relationship.

Our Upright Design

This four-footed design was further modified when some animals, in order to free up their forelimbs for digging, climbing, or flying, balanced themselves on their hind legs. This arrangement is demonstrated most dramatically in humans, who have fully exploited the strategy of coming up onto the hind limbs to a fully upright posture. This places the spine, as well as the muscles that support it, in a vertical arrangement. Perhaps most significantly, the head now sits, not in front of a horizontally-placed body (as in a dog), but on top of the vertically-oriented spine. Together, the head and spine comprise a crucial support structure upon which the muscles act to maintain the new upright posture. In the next chapter, we'll look at this system in depth.

In spite of the uniqueness of our upright design, however, we share a basic similarity with our evolutionary predecessors. The primitive spine and muscles first evolved to help fish move toward food. Sensory organs and their processing system, the brain, developed at the front end in order to take in information from the environment and to direct the appropriate motor activity. All body movements were organized in relation to the head and spine because all movement required locomotion in a forward direction, with the head leading.

In four-footed animals, this relationship of the head to the body is complicated by the fact that animals on land must first raise themselves off the ground in order to move forward. In humans, the head and spine are no longer arranged horizontally in line with movement. However, we must still organize ourselves against gravity with the head leading the body, and we still move largely in relation to sensory input from the eyes, ears, and nose. The head no longer leads in the direction of movement; it now leads us to go up to move in whatever direction we choose. Even in upright humans, the relationship of the head to the spine is the primary organizing principle in movement.

Upright Posture and the Evolution of Intelligence

Our upright posture, with our heads freely poised on top of our spines, renders us capable of a remarkable range of movements and skilled activities. With our arms freed from the task of bearing weight, we can grasp and manipulate objects, perform athletic feats, and generally explore the world with our hands. Our upright posture has led to increased visual capacity, the development of language and speech, and vastly enhanced cognitive abilities. It has also led to an expansion of the range of voluntary activity and of our consciousness. Our intelligence is directly related to our design.

Our upright design is also associated with fundamental changes in our nature. Many animals, such as dogs and cats, possess the ability to process information, to identify smells, to learn and remember—in other words, to think. In dogs and cats, however, the process of thinking is coupled to activity, reflecting a physical design in which information coming in through the head, such as the smell of food, is translated directly into movement aimed in the direction of the food.

This direct link between thought and action has all but disappeared in humans. We are capable of thinking quite independently of action. Our heads do not lead in the direction of movement but sit on top of our spines, making it possible to engage in activities in which thinking predominates over doing. We are able to stop and to contemplate the world and ourselves. Our upright design reflects our dual nature of being simultaneously rooted in the earth and dignified by our upright poise. Our evolving consciousness is ultimately made possible by our remarkable design. ■

2. Upright Support—Part I: The Extensors

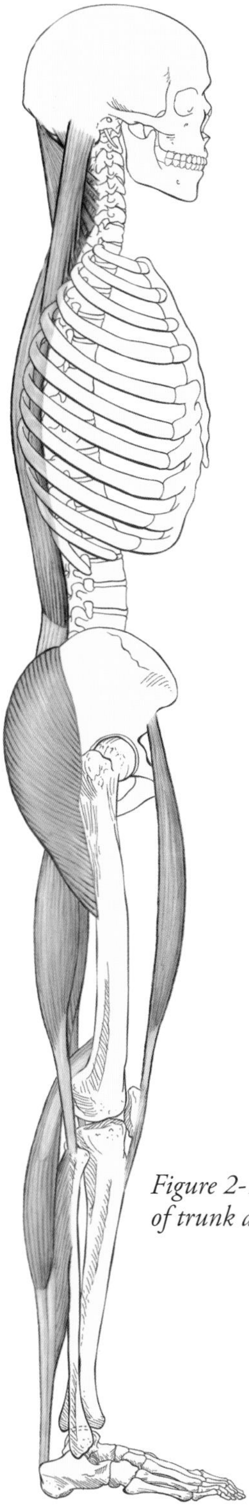

In the last chapter we looked at the basic function of muscle and bone, and how they work together to produce movement. In animals on land, muscle performs a dual function: it produces movement, and it maintains postural support against gravity. This postural function of muscle is so basic that it's impossible to speak of movement without reference to it; in order for any specific movement to take place, the muscular system as a whole must maintain the stability of the entire skeleton in relation to gravity. In humans, this feat must be accomplished in the fully upright posture, with the head balanced on top of a vertically-poised spine. Let's look now at our remarkable upright support system and how it works.

The Extensors

The primary muscles that support us against gravity are the extensors of the back and legs (Fig. 2-1). If you allow your body to go limp, you'll notice that as you begin to fall, your head, trunk, and knees buckle forward. In order to prevent this buckling, the extensor muscles, which lie primarily along the back of the body, must counteract this tendency by extending the legs and trunk (Fig. 2-2).

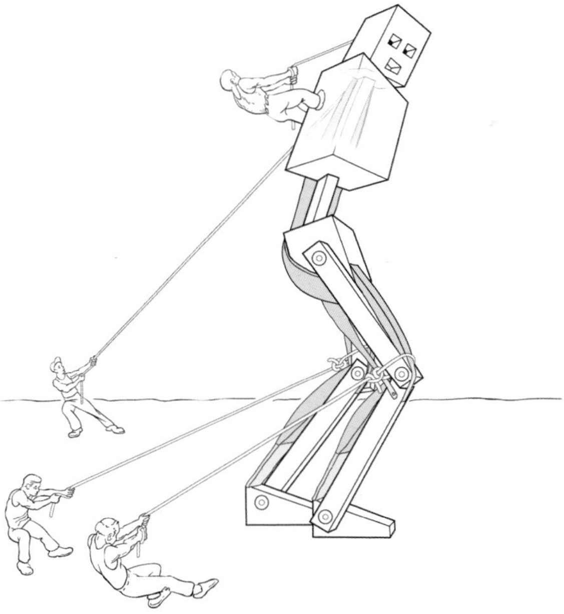

Figure 2-1. Extensors of trunk and legs.

Figure 2-2. Diagram showing where muscles are needed to keep a structure from falling down.

The word extensor comes from
the Latin *ex* + *tendere*, which
together mean "to stretch out."
In contrast, muscles that flex
joints are called "flexors," which
means "to bend." When we fall
forward, we flex at the joints;
in order to come up, we have to
use the extensors to counteract
this flexion. Thus there are two
muscle masses at work: flexors
along the front of the body
and extensors along the back.
The flexors bend the trunk and
limbs at the joints; the extensors
extend the limbs and support us
upright against gravity.

The most important extensors
are the muscles of the neck
and back. The back has five
layers of muscle. The most
superficial layers, which we'll
look at later, move the ribs and
shoulder blades and are not
directly involved in supporting
the trunk upright. It is the
two deepest layers, which lie
along the spine, that form
the extensors of the trunk.
The first and deepest layer is
comprised of a series of small
muscles running in between the
vertebrae of the spine along its
entire length, from the sacrum

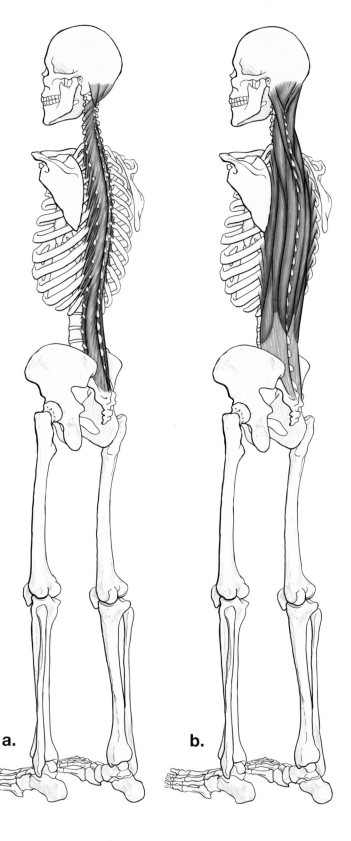

*Figure 2-3. Extensor
muscles of the back:
a. deep postural muscles;
b. erector spinae.*

a.

b.

to the occiput of the head. The second layer is comprised of long muscles which run vertically in meaty bundles up the length of the back from the sacrum to the base of the skull (Fig. 2-3).

Each of these layers serves a specific function. The smaller muscles of the back maintain the internal length and support of the spine. We often think of the spine as a singular, solid structure; in actuality, it consists of a series of separate vertebrae, with protrusions that form attachment points for ligaments and muscles. The ligaments bind the vertebrae together; the small muscles of the back, acting upon these attachments, help to straighten and elongate the spine (Fig. 2-3a). Additional muscles can be found lying along the front of the spine in the cervical and lumbar regions; these muscles work in conjunction with the extensor muscles to straighten the spinal curves (Fig. 2-4). So the deeper postural muscles in front and back work in tandem to support and elongate the spine itself.

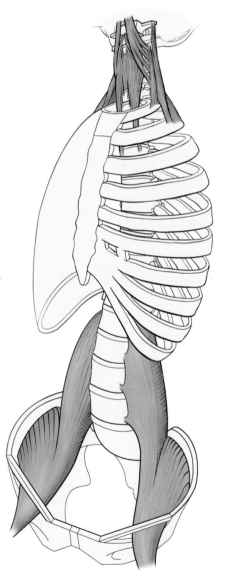

The second layer of muscles maintains the stability of the trunk as a whole in order to keep it from falling forward. When you are standing, and particularly if you are bending or carrying something, the weight of the rib cage and the organs in front of the spine drag the trunk down and forward. The large, long muscles of the back making up the second layer keep the trunk from buckling forward, which is why they are called the "erector spinae" muscles (Fig. 2-3b).

Figure 2-4. Muscles on the front of the spine that support the cervical and lumbar curves.

In addition to the trunk muscles, extensors along the legs and buttocks maintain the extension of the hips, knees, and ankles while standing. The muscles of the calves prevent the lower leg from buckling forward at the ankle. The muscles of the thigh prevent the knee from buckling. And the muscles of the buttocks stabilize the trunk at the hips. Together with the extensors of the neck and back, these muscles maintain erect posture by stabilizing the joints and keeping the body from buckling in response to gravity (Fig. 2-1).

If you look at Fig. 2-1, you'll see that the extensors of the thigh, unlike all the other extensors, run along the front of the body, not the back of it. This is because the knees buckle forward, and the primary muscles that must counteract this tendency are the quadriceps muscles of the thigh, which extend the leg at the knee. (These are the muscles that come into play when the doctor taps the tendon below the knee cap to elicit the classic knee-jerk response—the reflexive extension of the lower leg at the knee.) So all the extensors run along the back of the body except for the extensors of the leg at the knee, which lie along the front of the thigh.

Stretch Reflexes

To function effectively, it's critical that the extensor muscles know how much to tighten—and when. This is accomplished through receptors in the muscles which respond to stretch. When, for example, the knees buckle, the muscles of the thigh which extend the leg at the knee are stretched across the knee joint. The receptors in the muscle sense this increase in length and the muscle responds by contracting just enough to counteract it. These responses to stretch—or "stretch reflexes"—are occurring all the time at an unconscious level throughout the body. (The Greeks, noting this constant low-level activity in the muscles, called it "tonus" because of its resemblance to the way a stringed instrument's tone is determined by the stretch on its strings.)

Muscles are therefore responding constantly to external forces in order to stabilize the skeleton when we are standing or moving about. We think of muscles as holding us up, which of course they do; but it would be more accurate to say that once we are up off the ground, muscles keep us from falling down by sensing changes in length and adjusting constantly to these changes. This activity of postural muscles serves as the background against which all specific actions, like typing or throwing a ball, take place.

The Head and Spine

The most important postural muscles are those of the neck and back. As we've seen, two sets of muscles support the trunk—the small postural muscles connecting the vertebrae and the larger erector spinae muscles running from the sacrum up the entire length of the spine. Because these muscles attach to the base of the skull, they tend to pull the head back and increase the curvature of the spine, which interferes with upright support.

This is where the design of the skull and spine becomes so important. Though one might assume that the skull is exactly centered on top of the spine, this is not the case. In fact, the skull has more weight in front than in back, so that its natural tendency is to nod forward at the atlanto-occipital joint, the point where the skull articulates with the top vertebra of the spine (Fig. 2-5a). This forward weight exerts stretch on the extensor muscles at the back of the neck, which counteracts the tendency of these muscles to shorten or contract, reduces downward pressure of the skull on the spine, and has the effect of actually lengthening the spine (Fig. 2-5b).

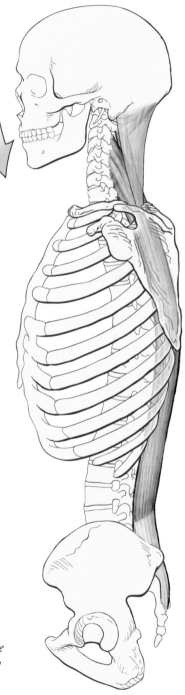

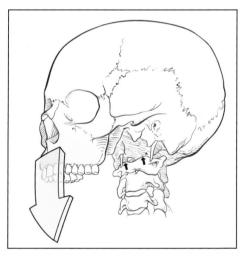

Figure 2-5a. Forward balance of the skull. The skull has more weight in front than in back.

Figure 2-5b. Head balance in relation to the extensors of neck and back. The forward weight of the head exerts stretch on the extensor muscles at the back of the neck and has the effect of actually lengthening the spine.

This lengthening of the spine is crucial to the functioning of the deeper postural muscles that support the spine. The vertebrae are cushioned by fluid-filled discs whose hydraulic properties impart buoyancy to the spine. Certain habitual postures such as pulling the head back or slumping tend to put pressure on the discs, which consequently lose buoyancy. The forward balance of the head at the atlanto-occipital joint reduces pressure on the spine, allowing the intervertebral discs to expand and restoring length to the spine. This increased lengthening of the spine exerts stretch on the small postural muscles, setting off stretch reflexes which further lengthen and support the spine.

The forward balance of the head on the spine is important to the extensor system in one other crucial respect. We've seen that the small postural muscles run between the vertebrae along the entire length of the spine (see Fig. 2-3). The uppermost of these muscles, which connect the first two vertebrae with the base of the skull (called the "sub-occipital muscles" because they lie just under the occiput), are crucial indicators of posture and balance in the body (Fig. 2-6). When we get out of bed in the morning or sit up from a slumped position—in other words, when the postural muscles have been disengaged and we need to right ourselves against gravity—it is the forward movement of the head on the spine that "tells" the deep postural muscles that we are about to assume an erect posture, setting off a series of "righting reflexes" that help support us against gravity.

If, as occurs in many people, the neck and trunk muscles are chronically shortened and the head is pulled back, the forward balance of the head on the spine is interfered with, and the deeper sub-occipital muscles at the base of the skull fail to register stretch. The postural system becomes confused, and we get stuck in postural attitudes that force the muscular system to work too hard and prevent the postural muscles from operating properly.

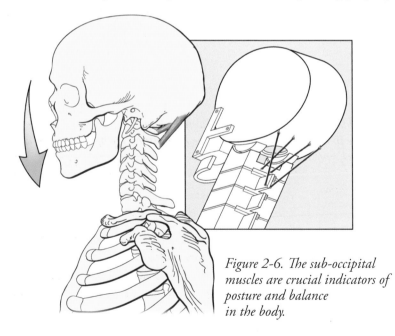

Figure 2-6. The sub-occipital muscles are crucial indicators of posture and balance in the body.

Muscles in the neck and trunk must be restored to their natural length so that the nodding forward of the head exerts stretch on the extensor muscles and signal when it's time to resume upright posture. We then experience a sense of lightness and buoyancy, of being supported against gravity without any sense of effort.

Head Balance

The importance of the head/spine relationship becomes easier to understand when you compare the human head/spine relationship with that of a four-footed animal such as a cat. Just as in humans, a cat's head and spine are designed to maintain length and tone in the back muscles. Obviously a cat's spine is horizontal, and the head, being in front of the spine, is able to drop down by its own weight and thereby counteract the pull of the neck muscles (Fig. 2-7a). In humans, this arrangement changes dramatically. Because the spine is vertical and the head sits on top of it, the head cannot exert stretch on the back muscles by dropping directly downward. The only way for nature to retain this stretch is for the head to sit off-center on top of the spine so that it tilts forward at the atlanto-occipital joint (Fig. 2-7b).

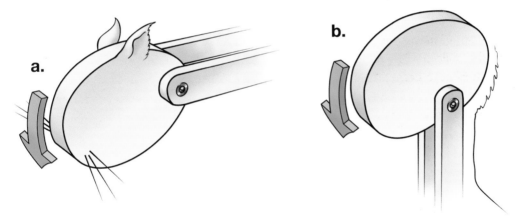

Figure 2-7a. Head balance in a cat. A cat's spine is horizontal, and the head, being in front of the spine, is able to drop down by its own weight. Figure 2-7b. Head balance in a human. Because the spine in humans is vertical and the head sits on top of it, the head cannot exert stretch on the back muscles by dropping directly downward. The only way for nature to retain this stretch is for the head to sit off-center on top of the spine so that it tilts forward at the atlanto-occipital joint.

Notice how much subtler this arrangement is than that of four-footed animals. The cat's head has no support from below and is simply pulled downward by gravity. This means that, no matter how strong the neck muscles are, the weight of the head easily counteracts the pull of these muscles, maintaining length and tone in the extensor muscles of the neck and back.

In humans, however, the head is supported from below and can counteract the pull of the neck muscles only by tilting delicately forward on the spine. In addition, the muscles of the neck and back run up and down, not sideways as in the cat. This means that the neck muscles pull directly downward, and that the forward balance of the head has to counteract this downward pull by exerting an upward pull directly opposing the force of gravity—a much more delicate mechanism than that of a four-footed animal, and for this reason more easily disturbed (Fig. 2-8). Were it not for this delicate arrangement, however, upright posture—and all the marvelous human traits that derived from it—would not be possible.

The forward balance of the head on the spine is thus integral to the human upright support system. Along with the structure of the spine itself, head balance is an essential component in maintaining stretch on the extensor muscles of the neck and back that keep us erect. These muscles are designed to keep us from falling over by maintaining the stability of the spine, trunk, and limbs; at the same time, they do not simply pull on bones but perform this function in the context of a marvelous system of counterbalancing skeletal forces that enables muscles to provide support against gravity with a minimum of effort. ■

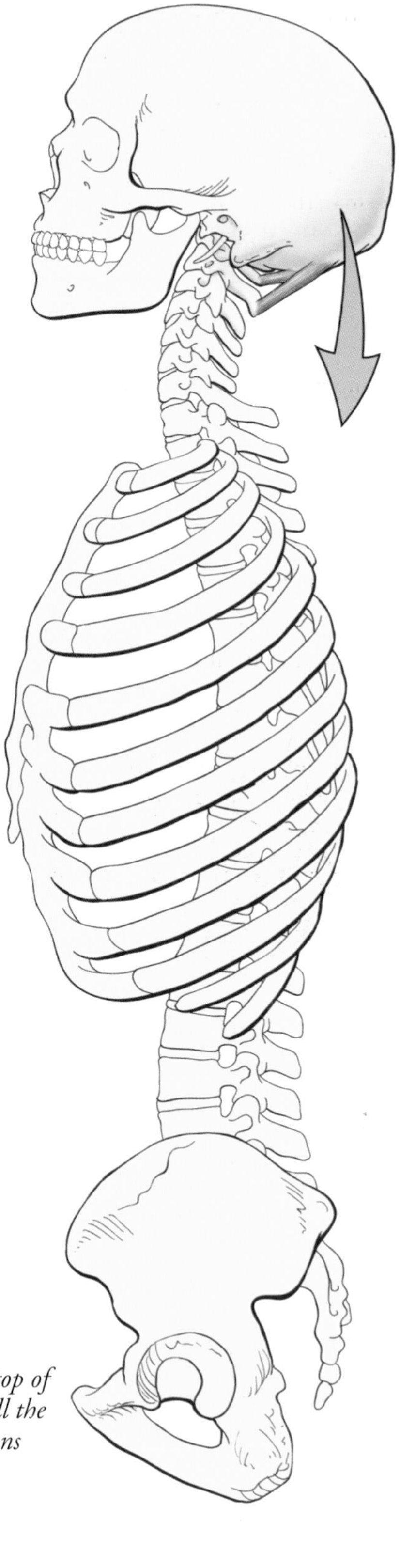

Figure 2-8. Disruption of head balance. Because the skull sits on top of the spine and the neck muscles pull the head back, head balance in humans can be easily disrupted.

3. Upright Support—Part II: The Flexors

In the last chapter we looked at the extensor muscles on the back of the body that support us against gravity by counteracting the tendency for the trunk and legs to buckle. The most important extensor muscles, as we saw, are the two layers of muscle lying closest to the spine. The deepest layer links all the bony projections of the vertebrae from sacrum to occiput, supporting the spine along its entire length. The second layer forms meaty bundles of muscles that travel in intervals up the spine from the sacrum to the skull. These muscles work most efficiently when the back is lengthened and when the head, which is balanced unevenly on top of the spine, falls forward and maintains stretch on the muscles of the neck and back. Let's look now at the flexors on the front of the body which oppose the extensors in back, and their crucial role in the upright support of the body.

Flexors and Our Basic Body Design

When we look in a very general way at the design of the body, one of its most obvious features is that the back is comprised almost entirely of the spine and its supporting muscles, and in front we have the rib cage and the internal organs. Intuitively this arrangement seems to make sense, but when asked why we are designed this way, most people would not be able to give a very clear answer. The explanation becomes obvious when we consider that, in a four-footed animal, the spine forms a kind of bridge which is suspended between the fore and hind limbs, and the rib cage and the internal organs which maintain basic life functions hang below the spine (Fig. 3-1).

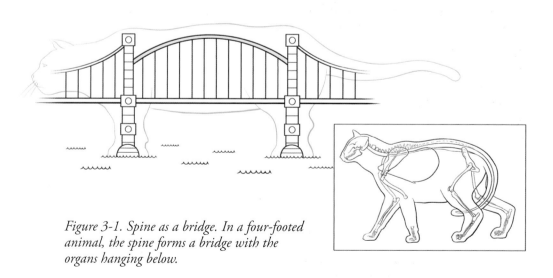

Figure 3-1. Spine as a bridge. In a four-footed animal, the spine forms a bridge with the organs hanging below.

15

When primates began to stand up on their hind limbs and raised the trunk to a more vertical position, the rib cage and organs which hung *below* the spine were now out in *front* (Fig. 3-2).

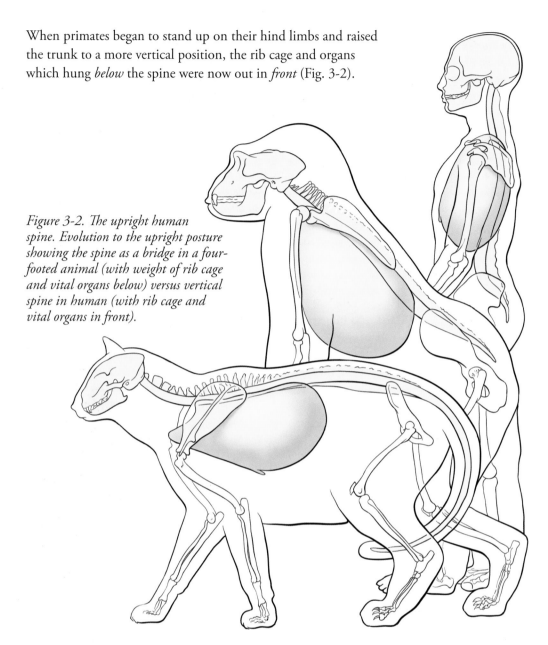

Figure 3-2. The upright human spine. Evolution to the upright posture showing the spine as a bridge in a four-footed animal (with weight of rib cage and vital organs below) versus vertical spine in human (with rib cage and vital organs in front).

This basic design feature explains a great deal when we consider the contrasting role of the flexors in front of the body and the extensors in back. If we had somehow pulled ourselves up directly from the ground, or built ourselves up from the ground like building blocks, we might suppose that the muscles in the front and back of our bodies would equally share the job of supporting us like guy wires on opposite sides of a tower. But humans didn't grow directly up from the ground; they stood up on their hind limbs by raising the trunk from the horizontal to the vertical. The main muscles that were needed to produce this action are in back, so that the main onus of postural support falls on the extensor muscles which prevent the legs from buckling and the trunk from falling forward (see Fig. 2-2).

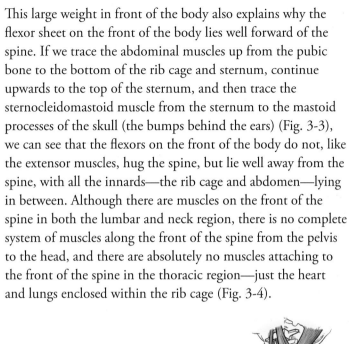

This large weight in front of the body also explains why the flexor sheet on the front of the body lies well forward of the spine. If we trace the abdominal muscles up from the pubic bone to the bottom of the rib cage and sternum, continue upwards to the top of the sternum, and then trace the sternocleidomastoid muscle from the sternum to the mastoid processes of the skull (the bumps behind the ears) (Fig. 3-3), we can see that the flexors on the front of the body do not, like the extensor muscles, hug the spine, but lie well away from the spine, with all the innards—the rib cage and abdomen—lying in between. Although there are muscles on the front of the spine in both the lumbar and neck region, there is no complete system of muscles along the front of the spine from the pelvis to the head, and there are absolutely no muscles attaching to the front of the spine in the thoracic region—just the heart and lungs enclosed within the rib cage (Fig. 3-4).

Figure 3-3. Flexor muscles on the front of the body: abdominals and sternocleidomastoid muscle.

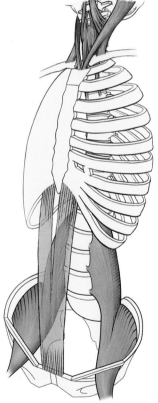

Figure 3-4. Flexor muscles on the front of the spine are in cervical and lumbar regions only.

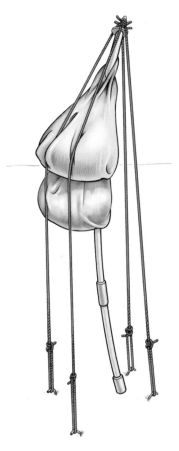

This arrangement becomes clearer if you think of a tent-pole supported by guy wires, with bags or appendages hanging from one side of the tent pole (which in humans is the front). A number of guy wires must support the "back" of the tent pole to keep it from falling over, but in front, the guy wires can't hug the tent pole but must run along the outside of the bags. Now of course our spines are certainly not tent-poles, but our back muscles, like the guy wires on the back of the tent pole, do work closely with the spine to maintain upright posture. But because there is a large mass of stuff in front—the rib cage and all the internal organs—the flexors on the front of the body run along the outside of these structures (Fig. 3-5).

I should add that the abdominal muscles that run vertically up to the sternum are not the only flexors on the front of the body. There are also flexors that wrap around the trunk at an oblique angle, so that the rib cage and abdomen are encircled by muscles running around it in spirals. We'll look at these muscles in more depth later when we discuss breathing and the spiral musculature. For our present purposes, however, it is easiest to think of the flexors as a direct line of muscles running up the front of the body from the pubic bone to the mastoid process of the skull.

Figure 3-5. Tent pole and guy wires.

At the most obvious level, these muscles help to flex the trunk and neck, as when we are lying on our backs and do a sit-up. They also help to stabilize the trunk, as anyone who's had abdominal surgery knows. If your abdominal muscles are sore or injured and cannot contract properly, it is difficult to move or even to stand upright, since these actions require quite a lot of muscular tone and support to stabilize the trunk. Tonus in the abdominal muscles also helps to maintain pressure on the abdominal contents, which in turn adds support to the trunk. In this sense, the flexors in the front of the body counterbalance the extensors in back.

The Suspensory Function of the Flexors

But the flexors have another very important function. Being upright, as we saw earlier, makes a number of unique demands on the human body. The back muscles must maintain the extension of the spine and trunk. The head balances unevenly atop the vertically-placed spine. The spine itself has developed several curves to help support upright posture. It must also be able to absorb shock and resist compression in order to support the weight of the body, to maintain the length of the trunk, and to work with muscles to create lengthened support against gravity.

But what about the weight in front of the body? Here we have a different set of problems. The rib cage, which hangs down in front, tends to drop, as well as the abdominal contents below the rib cage. The structures of the jaw, the throat, and the larynx, which are all suspended from the skull, tend to pull downward on the skull and create an additional drag in front of the body. Even further drag is added when we

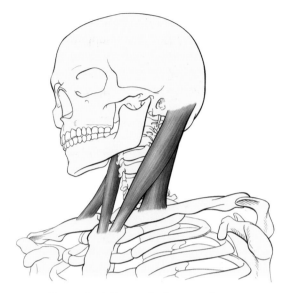

Figure 3-6. Sternocleidomastoid muscles supporting the rib cage.

use our arms or carry weight in front of us, which contributes to the common tendency of humans living in sedentary conditions to pull down and collapse in front. This reduces the volume of the chest and abdomen, interferes with breathing, and presses on the gut, which tends to sag with age.

This is where the flexors come in. We saw a moment ago that the musculature along the front of the body ultimately attaches to the skull via the sternocleidomastoid muscle, which originates at the sternum and clavicles and attaches to the mastoid processes. This means that the rib cage is, in a sense, suspended from the head by the sternocleidomastoid muscle (Fig. 3-6). This is also true, as we shall see in Chapter Five, of the shoulder girdle, which is suspended from above by muscles; but the point is that the rib cage and, in fact, the entire front of the body, which tends to sag downward, is supported from above by the flexor muscles on the front of the body which attach to the head. If we are not interfering with this support by habitually collapsing or drawing ourselves down in front, the flexors are able to maintain the length and volume of the body in front that form a key component of our upright posture.

Clearly we can see that these muscles in front do not support the body in the same way the back does. Because it has so much weight in front, the trunk is inherently unstable and tends to fall forward; the muscles in back work with the spine to maintain the erect posture. But the muscles in front have a very different function: they support the structures hanging in front of the body, which are suspended from the skull. When the flexors are working properly, they maintain tensile length and muscular tone in the front of the body which counteracts the extensors in back. So in contrast to the spine, which resists compression in order to bear weight and to maintain the structural length of the trunk, the flexors on the front of the body comprise a tensile structure for suspending the ribs and maintaining the support of the front of the body.

This gives us a more complete picture of what is involved in achieving a lengthened support of the body. Elasticity and stretch on the muscles of the neck and back are required in order for the extensors to function efficiently. But it is just as crucial that the weight of the structures in front—throat, rib cage, and innards—does not compromise the length and volume of the trunk, or cause the back to overwork. In order for this to happen, the flexors and rib cage must release and undo into length, which in turn allows the extensors to do their job so that the trunk can naturally lengthen and expand in response to gravity.

Front Length and Head Balance

Let us look at a final and crucial factor governing the role of the flexors in upright balance. We saw a moment ago that the jaw, throat, and larynx are suspended from the skull and tend to drag it down—that is, they flex the skull. We might attribute the same tendency to the flexors on the front of the body, since the extensors retract the head and the flexors would appear to produce the opposite effect. But in fact it doesn't work this way. If you look closely at the sternocleidomastoid muscle, which is the key neck muscle connecting the flexor sheet on the front of the body to the head, you'll see that its point of attachment at the mastoid process of the skull is slightly behind the atlanto-occipital joint, the point at which the skull balances on the spine. This means that, although the sternocleidomastoid muscle will tend to drag the neck or upper spine forward, it will actually pull the head back in relation to the spine (Fig. 3-7). This pull becomes even more accentuated when we collapse or draw ourselves down in front, which drags upon the neck and upper spinal column, rotates the mastoid process forward, and thus increases the drag of the sternocleidomastoid muscle on the head. In order to counter this tendency and to maintain upward support, the head must balance forward on top of the

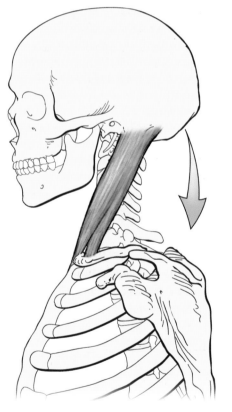

Figure 3-7. Backward pull of sternocleidomastoid muscle on head.

spine so that, instead of dragging down upon the head, the rib cage and abdomen are suspended from above.

Once again we find that the balance of the head is a key organizing factor governing the working of the muscular system. The forward balance of the head is crucial to the lengthened working of the back muscles, but it is equally crucial to the length and support of the body in front. Because the front of the body is suspended from the head and, as we've seen, paradoxically tends to pull it back, the head must be balanced forward in order to maintain front length as well. When it comes to the various elements involved in musculoskeletal support, all paths lead to Rome—the organizing principle of the relation of the head to the trunk which is so crucial to the muscle systems that support us against gravity (Fig. 3-8).

To summarize, the spine, which bears weight, is supported by close-lying extensor muscles which maintain extension of the spine and support the trunk. In the human upright posture, the throat, rib cage, and internal organs lie in front of the spine and tend to create a downward drag on the body. Because these structures are largely suspended from flexors attaching to the skull, a key role of these muscles is to maintain natural length or tensile support along the front of the body, counteracting this downward pull in front. And because these flexors attach to a point on the skull just behind its point of balance, front length ultimately depends on the forward and up direction of the head.

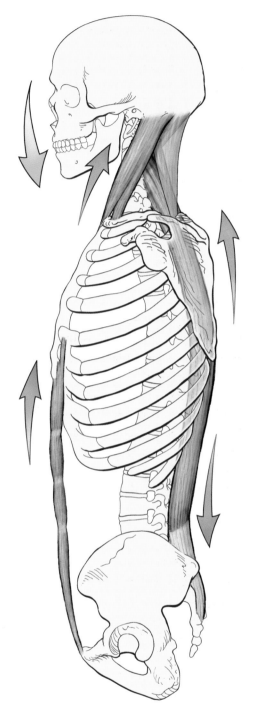

Figure 3-8. Head Balance. The forward balance of the head is crucial to the lengthened working of the back muscles, but it is equally crucial to the length and support of the body in front.

The natural balance of the head, however, is not a position and cannot be established through direct effort. Because we are capable of voluntarily altering the position of the head and have been taught to have good posture, it is tempting to think that we can achieve desirable posture by deliberately correcting the position of the head and rib cage. But think about what this actually means in practice. Because the flexors in front of the body actually have the effect of pulling back the head, fixing the head in this manner actually prevents the head from going up by keeping us shortened in front. If we want to achieve true lengthened support of the trunk, we must not put the head forward and down but instead allow it to go up in such a way that the body can lengthen in front as well as in back. We must remember that head balance is not a goal in itself but a natural condition of the entire muscular system in which the trunk is able to regain flexibility and expansion. Allowing the head to go up by not interfering with the length in front of the body is a key component of this process. ■

4. Upright Support—Part III: The Spine

In the last chapter we looked at the spine and the muscles along the front and back of the body which maintain the upright support of the trunk. Let's take a closer look now at the spine itself, its remarkable design, and its specific contributions to our upright support.

The Central Column

The spine, or backbone, is the central bony structure of the body upon which muscles act to support us against gravity and to produce movement. Many exercise and relaxation systems emphasize the role of muscles and underestimate the importance of bones in general and the spine in particular to the study of movement and muscles. But it is important to remember that, in order for us to be supported against gravity and for movement to take place, muscles need a solid structure to act upon. In all vertebrates, the spine is the primary bony structure, and it is supported and acted upon by a complex network of muscles.

The spine, or backbone, is a flexible column formed by the vertebrae and the intervertebral discs (the word "vertebra" is from *vertere*, which means "to turn"). There are thirty-three vertebrae in all: seven in the cervical (neck) region, twelve in the thoracic (chest) region, five in the lumber region, five in the sacral (pelvic) region, and four in the coccygeal (tailbone) region. The sacral and coccygeal vertebrae are fused together to form the sacrum and coccyx, so that for all intents and purposes the spine consists of twenty-four moveable vertebrae, plus the sacrum and tailbone (Fig. 4-1).

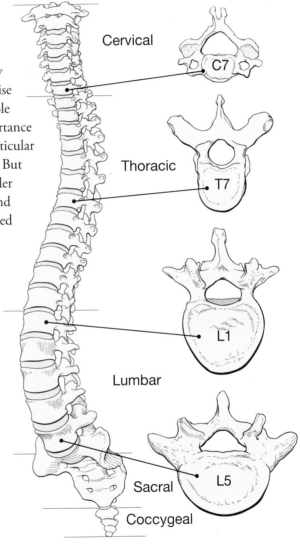

Cervical

C7

Thoracic

T7

L1

Lumbar

L5

Sacral

Coccygeal

Figure 4-1. The spine consists of twenty-four movable vertebrae, plus the sacrum and tailbone.

23

The main purpose of the spine is to bear weight and to provide a support structure for muscles to act upon in producing upright balance and movement. Each vertebra has two parts. The front part, called the "body" or "centrum," is round and forms a weight-bearing column of bony segments stacked on top of each other with intervertebral discs in between (Fig. 4-2). The intervertebral discs are resilient and pliable structures designed to absorb shock as well as to allow twisting and bending of the spine; together with the vertebral bodies, they form a strong yet flexible column for supporting the head and trunk. The vertebral bodies and the intervertebral discs are smaller at the top and get much larger and stronger at the bottom, where they must support greater weight.

The back part of the vertebra, called the "arch," has several functions (Fig. 4-2). First, flattened sections on the arch articulate with corresponding surfaces on the vertebrae above and below to form joints that give the spine stability while still making it possible for it to bend and twist. Second, protruding sections of the arch, called "processes," form attachments for muscles and ligaments which act upon and support the spine. Finally, the entire arch forms a hole, or canal, just behind the body of the vertebra, which protects the spinal cord running through it. Branches of the spinal cord project laterally out of small holes between the vertebrae, extending peripheral nerves to the trunk and limbs.

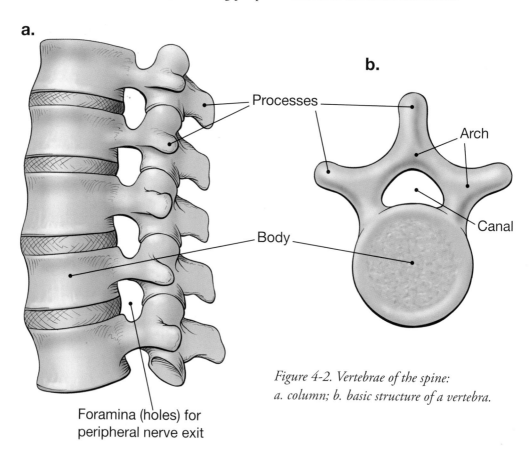

a.

b.

Processes

Arch

Body

Canal

Foramina (holes) for peripheral nerve exit

Figure 4-2. Vertebrae of the spine: a. column; b. basic structure of a vertebra.

Origins of the Human Spine

But how did the spine become the way it is, with all its intricacies and protrusions? As we saw in Chapter One, the spine first evolved in fish to prevent the body from telescoping when it flexed its body from side to side (see Fig. 1-1). Just above this primitive spine, called the "notochord," ran a central nerve which supplied the muscles and organs throughout the body (Fig. 4-3).

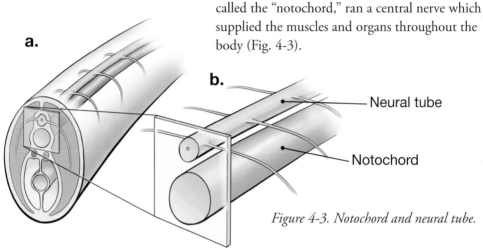

Figure 4-3. Notochord and neural tube.

In some species of fish, bone began to form in segments around the nerve cord, forming a "neural arch" that protected the nerve cord (Fig. 4-4a). The notochord, too, began to ossify in segments and joined with the forming arches, so that it was soon replaced by a series of bony vertebrae with intervertebral discs in between (Fig. 4-4b).

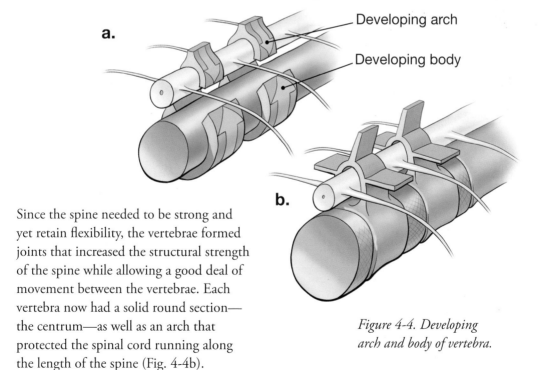

Since the spine needed to be strong and yet retain flexibility, the vertebrae formed joints that increased the structural strength of the spine while allowing a good deal of movement between the vertebrae. Each vertebra now had a solid round section—the centrum—as well as an arch that protected the spinal cord running along the length of the spine (Fig. 4-4b).

Figure 4-4. Developing arch and body of vertebra.

In this way, the notochord was replaced by a flexible spinal column that could be acted upon by muscles to produce movement; the only remnant of the notochord in the human spine is the viscous central portion of the intervertebral disc, called the *nucleus pulposa*. The spine was now a strong yet flexible structure that protected the spinal cord and, at the same time, provided sturdy attachments for muscles—a very logical design once you look at it from the point of view of its evolution and function.

Upright Posture and the Spinal Curves

Note that, in its original form, the spine had nothing to do with support *per se*; it simply provided a flexible beam to support the body and to provide attachments for muscles. Accordingly, a fish's spine, which consists only of a trunk and tail section, is rather straight and undifferentiated, with a head at one end and a tail at the other (Fig. 4-5a). In animals that come onto land, the design of the spine changes considerably. In order to move on land, reptiles must be able to get the body up off the ground by supporting themselves on their limbs. The spine then begins to function like a bridge between the fore and hind limbs with the ribs and major organs suspended beneath it (Fig. 4-5b); this curve of the spine defines the thoracic region. Also, the pelvic bones form attachments to the spine so that force from the legs can be directly transmitted to the trunk; this defines the sacral region of the spine (see Fig. 7-4a on page 52). In reptiles that move close to the ground, the spine is only mildly curved. Since four-footed mammals such as dogs and cats stand higher off the ground, the spine developed a broad curve which supports the body over the fore and hind limbs, and a compensating curve at the neck so that the head can be held at the same height as the body, or higher. The spine now has: a curve at the neck, or cervical region; a broad curve of the back, or thoracic region; a sacral region where the pelvis connects with the spine; a lumbar region between the ribs and sacrum; and a tail (Fig. 4-5c).

In apes, the trunk is brought more vertically over the pelvis (Fig. 4-5d); although still somewhat four-footed, chimpanzees and gorillas are able to walk on two legs and, when they sit on their haunches, to use their freed upper limbs to manipulate objects. In the upright human posture, the trunk is entirely up-ended so that the head sits directly on top of an erect spine. Instead of functioning as a bridge, the central column of the spine—the vertebral bodies and the intervertebral discs—becomes a weight-bearing, compression-resistant column for the vertically-poised trunk (Fig. 4-5e). The upper spinal column is narrow and lightweight because it has only to bear the relatively small weight of the head; it thickens toward the bottom, where it bears the weight of the entire trunk. The thoracic curve is retained as the major curve of the spine and the cervical curve now accommodates the head, which balances on the top vertebra, the atlas. At the sacrum, the vertebrae become fused to support the pelvic girdle; below it, the coccyx is the only remnant of our vestigial tail (see Fig. 4-1).

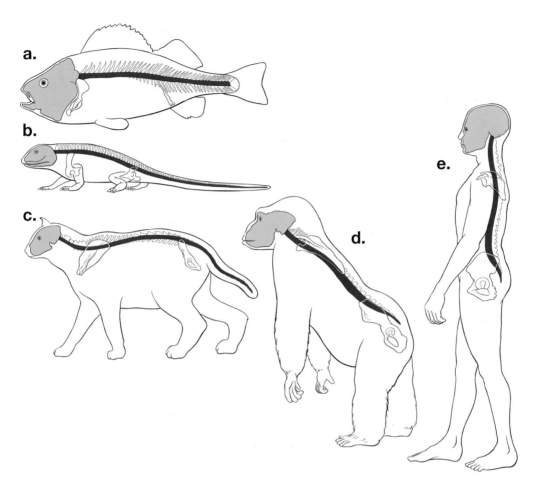

Figure 4-5. Evolutionary development of the spine: a. fish; b. reptile; c. cat; d. gorilla; e. human.

Notice that the spine now becomes oriented to movement in a new way. We saw in the case of marine animals that the spine flexes from side to side to produce locomotion through the water. This design is retained in many amphibians and lizards that advance their sprawled limbs by flexing the body from side to side. In mammals such as horses and cats, however, this design changes drastically. The limbs are brought under the body and the legs are oriented to convey propulsive thrust directly to the spine and trunk. By coiling the thoracic curve of the spine while gathering their legs underneath them and then uncoiling the spine like a spring when pushing off with the hind legs, the spine now flexes, not side to side as in a fish or reptile, but front to back. This front-to-back flexion remains a defining trait of upright human posture, making it possible for us to curl into a fetal position, to crouch and squat, and to slump when we are sitting carelessly.

Another major change in the human spine is the development of independent movement of the head due to alterations in the vertebrae of the neck. In a fish, the entire body swings from side to side; the head has no freedom of movement independently of the spine. In land animals, the vertebrae of the neck become modified so that the head can hinge up and down at the atlas as well as rotate freely; in some animals, the neck becomes completely movable so that it functions somewhat like a limb that can move the head independently of the trunk. In humans, the neck remains quite flexible and the head, which sits on top of the spine, is capable of nodding up and down and rotating. But because the spine is vertically poised, the head now rotates on a vertical axis, giving us a greatly expanded visual field (see Fig. 12-2 on page 88).

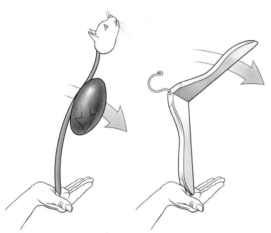

Figure 4-6. The thoracic curve in a four-footed animal can't support upright posture.

Perhaps the biggest change in the design of the human spine, however, is the addition of a lumbar curve. With only one broad thoracic curve, four-footed animals cannot support themselves easily on two legs because they're so heavily weighted in front (Fig. 4-6). In order to come upright onto two feet, primates began to develop a compensating curve in the lumbar region to counterbalance the thoracic curve and the forward tilt of the pelvis.

The result, in humans, is four curves—cervical, thoracic, lumbar, and sacral (two inner ones balancing two outer ones) —which provide a flexible, balanced column that can support fully upright posture (Fig. 4-7).

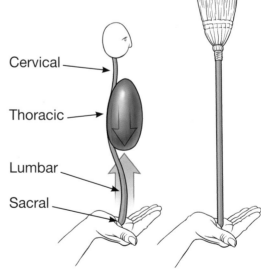

Figure 4-7. The balanced curves in the human spine are designed to support upright posture.

This means that the curves of the spine aren't incidental to upright posture but an integral part of it. The lumbar curve of the spine is essential to upright posture, and humans are the only primate with a fully-developed lumbar curve that balances the thoracic curve of the spine. That curve—along with our many other design features—makes us the only truly upright creature in the animal kingdom, completely freeing our upper limbs and making possible our distinctively human striding gait.

The Spine as Lengthening Device

The final elements that support the vertically-poised spine, of course, are ligaments and muscles. We've seen that the spine is bound together by a number of short ligaments that form a truss-work between the vertebrae, as well as long ligaments that bind the entire spine into one unit. These ligaments are matched by a number of small muscles that support the vertebrae from the sacrum up to the occiput of the head. As we've seen, these muscles do not simply pull on the vertebrae but are stretched between the processes of the vertebrae and then respond to this stretch by maintaining constant tone.

In order for this to occur, however, the spine must maintain its internal length. The intervertebral discs are made up of tough, fibrous outer shells encasing a nucleus filled with fluid. If the discs are subjected to constant pressure they lose resiliency, which accounts for the variability in height that can occur from morning to night. With age, the discs gradually lose their elasticity and ability to absorb moisture, which accounts in part for loss of height in old age. When the spine and its supporting muscles are functioning properly, however, these discs impart length and buoyancy to the spine and the vertebrae act as spacers for the small muscles of the back, maintaining the elasticity and stretch essential to their optimal functioning.

Working in conjunction with its supporting muscles, then, the spine acts as a lengthening device to support upright posture. The curves of the spine are built into its structural design, but without the dynamic action of the extensor muscles, these curves become exaggerated and we lose the internal length and support required for balanced upright posture. When this happens, we develop postural distortions, overwork various muscles groups, and place strain on the ligaments and undue pressure on the discs and bones. The only thing that can prevent this is the active support of postural muscles that maintain the length of the spine. We think of posture as either "good" or "bad," as if the curves of the spine are simply a matter of shape or degree. But lengthening is part of our inherent design; we are *meant* to lengthen as part of how the spine and muscular system are designed to keep us upright.

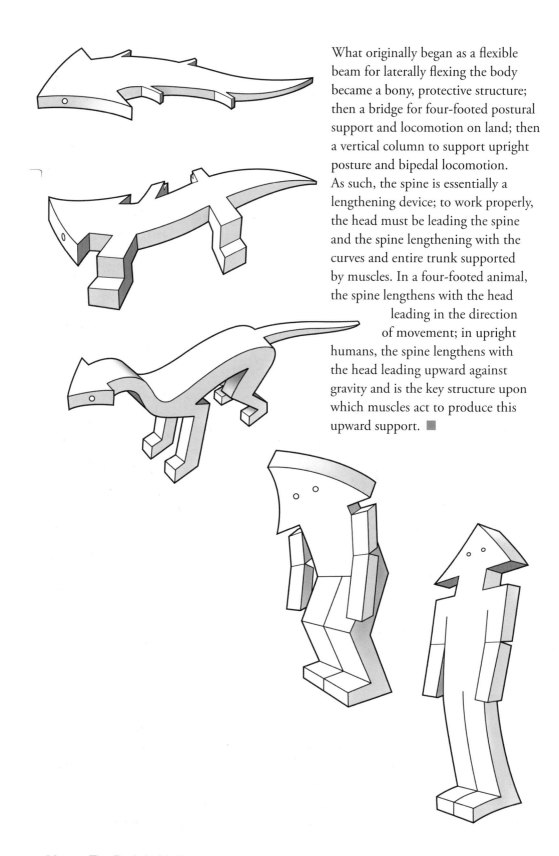

What originally began as a flexible
beam for laterally flexing the body
became a bony, protective structure;
then a bridge for four-footed postural
support and locomotion on land; then
a vertical column to support upright
posture and bipedal locomotion.
As such, the spine is essentially a
lengthening device; to work properly,
the head must be leading the spine
and the spine lengthening with the
curves and entire trunk supported
by muscles. In a four-footed animal,
the spine lengthens with the head
leading in the direction
of movement; in upright
humans, the spine lengthens with
the head leading upward against
gravity and is the key structure upon
which muscles act to produce this
upward support. ▪

5. The Shoulder Girdle

In the last several chapters we looked at the major systems that support the trunk in the upright posture, including the extensors, the flexors, and the spine. Let's turn now to the shoulder girdle.

The Mobile Cross-Piece

Put simply, the shoulder girdle is a support structure for the arm. If you think of the arm as a system of levers for moving the hand, which in turn grasps and manipulates objects, then the shoulder girdle is the crosspiece for the arm levers. Since the ribs are rather wide at the chest, it appears that the arm hangs from the rib cage. But the upper rib cage is in fact very narrow, and the arm is not attached directly to the rib cage but hangs from the shoulder girdle, which gives breadth to the upper torso. And although the shoulder girdle is linked into the trunk with a number of powerful muscles, it is actually suspended above the ribs and moves quite independently of the trunk, thus providing a support structure for the levers of the arm that is not only powerful, but highly mobile.

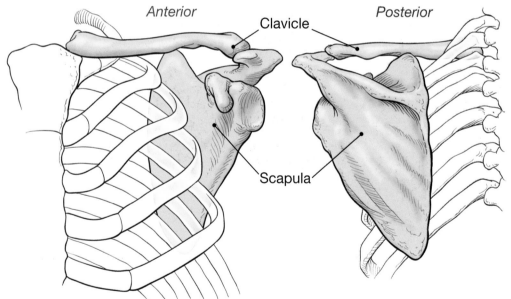

Figure 5-1. The shoulder girdle.

The shoulder girdle is made up of two bones: the clavicle, or collar bone, and the scapula, or shoulder blade (Fig. 5-1). At first glance it's hard to imagine how the shoulder acquired its unusual design. However, if you look at this structure from the point of view of what it does, it begins to make perfect sense. If you were designing a robot and wanted to give it arms, or long levers, with a hand at the end so that it could grasp things, you would probably extend the arm levers from a socket attached to the body of the robot. That's precisely what the scapula is: a socket for the head of the humerus, the long bone of the upper arm. Because the scapula must be firmly anchored to the body, it needs to function as more than just a socket; it must have sufficient surface area so that it can be firmly tied into the trunk with muscles—particularly in back, where it needs the most support. The scapula, then, is a broad, flat bone situated in back, with a shallow socket for the shoulder joint and various protrusions that provide attachment points for muscles to anchor it in place (Fig. 5-1).

But why isn't the shoulder a simple crosspiece, with a socket on each end for the upper arm bones? There are several reasons: First, if the crosspiece were fixed in place, the arm wouldn't be very mobile. If you create a yoke-like crosspiece for the shoulder joints with sockets in each end, the range of movement of a lever extending from a ball in each socket would be quite limited (Fig. 5-2a). In order for the arm to be truly mobile, the socket itself —in other words, the scapula—needs to be movable (Fig. 5-2b). This makes it possible not only to move the arm in relation to the scapula, but the scapula in relation to the body (Fig. 5-2c).

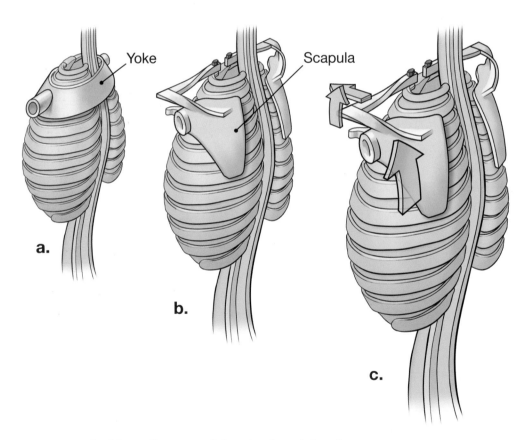

Figure 5-2. Shoulder girdle: a. immobile socket; b. mobile socket; c. mobile socket with arrows showing added range of motion.

Movement of the scapula is crucial to the functional usefulness of the arm. Over a third of the range of motion of the arm comes from the movement of the scapula; without the assistance of this mobile socket, the arm would not be able to perform many of its most important functions.

Second, the arm needs to be able to move powerfully and vigorously, which is why the scapula and upper arm are tied into the trunk by powerful muscles along the entire length of the spine and on both the front and back of the trunk (Figs. 5-3 and 5-8). If the socket of the arm were fixed, the arm wouldn't derive any strength from the torso; it would only swing rather pathetically from the shoulder. But the shoulder and arm are acted upon by the broad muscles of the chest and the entire back, making it possible to perform the most powerful swinging, throwing, and climbing motions.

Since the action of muscles moving the shoulder girdle adds power and force to the action of the arms, the arms must also be able to move vigorously and sustain impact without disturbing the trunk and, as we'll see in a moment, without limiting the movement and freedom of the ribs. For this reason, the scapula is not directly attached to the spine or ribs but suspended entirely within this network of muscles. Imagine what would happen if every time we threw a ball or supported weight on our arms the force of the arm movement violently jolted the ribs. Because the shoulder girdle is attached to the skeleton only at the sternum, force from the arm is absorbed by the network of muscles supporting the scapula.

We saw earlier that the extensor muscles, which run vertically along the length of the back, comprise the two deepest layers of back muscles. In contrast, the muscles that support and move the scapulae and humerus lie on top of the deeper

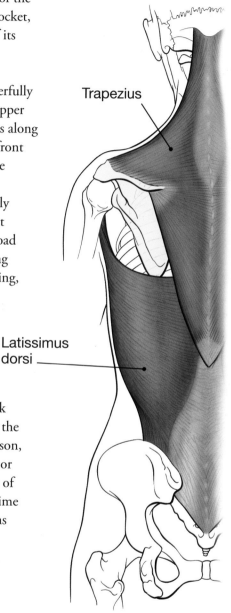

Trapezius

Latissimus dorsi

Figure 5-3. Muscles from entire length of spine converging into shoulder (superficial or fifth layer).

layers and run more obliquely, comprising the outer (fourth and fifth) layers of back muscles. The fourth layer supports and moves the scapulae (Fig. 5-4); the superficial fifth layer, which consists of the latissimus dorsi and trapezius muscles, spreads out in a large sheet that covers practically the entire back and attaches to both the scapulae and upper arms (see Fig. 5-3). It is these superficial layers of back muscles that give us the ability to move the scapulae and arms in such powerful and sweeping movements.

Precisely because the shoulder girdle is so mobile, however, it must also be possible to anchor it in place, as when we support the weight of our bodies on our arms, hang from a branch, or carry a heavy object. Using the arms requires that we be able to both move and stabilize the scapulae, often in combination.

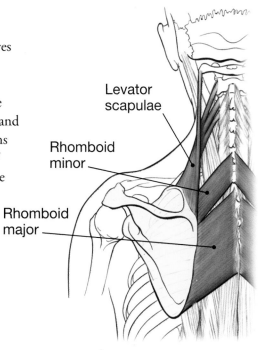

Levator scapulae

Rhomboid minor

Rhomboid major

Figure 5-4. Muscles moving the scapula (the fourth layer).

The Yard-Arm

For the scapula to be this versatile, however, it needs a kind of strut, or yard-arm, to anchor the scapula at a fixed distance from the body and limit its range of motion. This helps the shoulder to absorb shock while keeping the shoulder joint from being pulled into or away from the body. That yard-arm is the clavicle, which permits the scapula a broad range of motion while anchoring it to the sternum (Fig. 5-1). This makes it possible to maintain the stability of the shoulder while moving the arm quite vigorously, and to support the weight of the body when we hang from our arms, as our tree-dwelling ancestors did quite regularly.

In summary, the scapula functions as a movable joint for the arm, the clavicle serves as a yard-arm for the scapula, and the scapula moves freely on the ribs around the pivoting arm of the clavicle in order to provide added mobility and power to the arms. This entire bony structure provides attachments for muscles that anchor and move it with incredible efficiency while suspending it freely above the rib cage, to which it's connected only at the sternum—altogether an amazingly versatile mechanism.

From Fins to Limbs

A brief look at the evolution of the shoulder girdle will help to further clarify why our arms are designed the way they are. A reptile uses its limbs as levers in order to move along the ground. These limbs evolved from the pectoral and pelvic fins of certain species of fish that were able to "crawl" in the shallows, began to come onto land, and evolved a complex musculature for support and locomotion on four legs (Fig. 5-5). Most reptiles move with their bellies close to the ground and limbs sprawled to the sides. In mammals, the legs are brought more directly underneath the body, making it possible to move more quickly and efficiently. Certain tree-dwelling primates developed prehensile limbs and tails and a partially upright posture that gave them the ability to walk on their hind legs, thus freeing their highly developed forelimbs to function as arms.

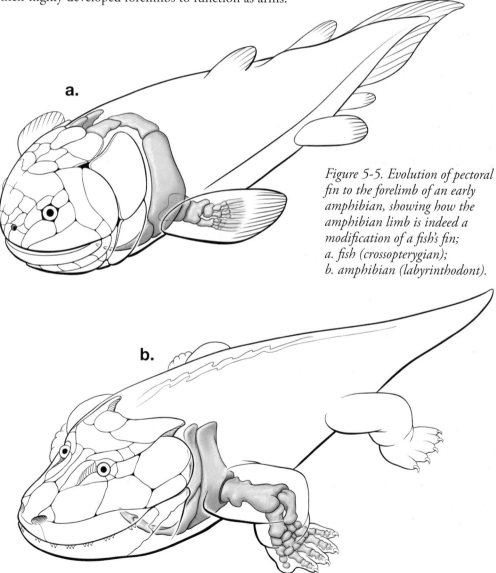

Figure 5-5. Evolution of pectoral fin to the forelimb of an early amphibian, showing how the amphibian limb is indeed a modification of a fish's fin; a. fish (crossopterygian); b. amphibian (labyrinthodont).

In the most advanced of these primates, the forelimbs became quite powerful and highly mobile, which allowed not just climbing and swinging but even the primitive use of tools. Then came the first fully upright hominids, whose arms and hands were entirely emancipated from their weight-bearing function and could be used solely for manipulation—a dramatic evolutionary step which led to increasing control over the environment and a tremendous leap in the evolution of the brain.

The erect posture completely altered the design of the shoulder girdle. Muscles along the entire length of the spine and trunk converged into the shoulder, imparting both range and power to the movement of the arms (Fig. 5-3). From the exceedingly limited and circumscribed movements of our four-footed ancestors, the human shoulder girdle became the most highly mobile joint in the body, permitting the arm a sweeping range of movement and giving the hands much greater control.

The human shoulder girdle thus became ideally suited as a mobile support structure for the arms, which in turn are capable of bringing food to the mouth, lifting and manipulating objects, and touching and exploring the world. The arm has other functions as well, including support, throwing, fighting, and climbing—many of which we can see developed to their highest perfection in dance, theater, sports, and the martial arts. For these and other purposes, the shoulder girdle is a remarkable instrument for permitting a wide range of powerful and subtle movements. In exchange for this mobility, the shoulder has become much less stable than the hips, which now must bear the full weight of the body.

The Floating Shoulder Girdle

In order to function properly, however, the shoulder girdle must participate in the lengthened support of the trunk. In Chapter Two, we saw how the front of the body is suspended from above by muscles. In the same way, the shoulder girdle is suspended by the trapezius and levator scapulae muscles in back and the sternocleidomastoid muscle in front (Fig. 5-6), which enable it to "float" above the rib cage so that it can be moved freely and can function independently of the ribs.

This suspensory support of the shoulder girdle is directly related to the muscles supporting the trunk. So long as the shoulders and arms do not squeeze down upon the rib cage and the extensor and flexor muscles on the front and back of the body are maintaining the full length of the trunk, the chest and shoulders will remain open and the shoulder girdle will remain lightly supported above the rib cage. With this support coming from the trunk, it is possible to use the arms for extended periods, while engaged in even the most demanding tasks, without any sense of undue effort or strain.

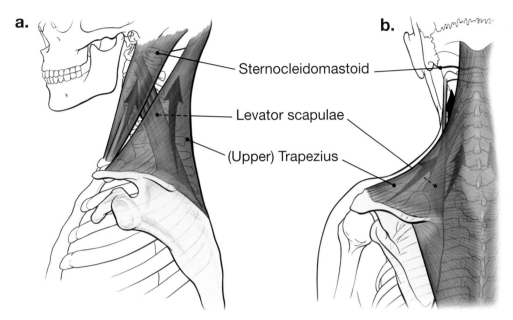

a. Sternocleidomastoid

Levator scapulae

(Upper) Trapezius

b.

Figure 5-6. Suspensory muscles of the shoulder girdle: a. lateral view; b. posterior view.

The universal tendency in using the arms, however, is to collapse and shorten the body in front, to drop the arms so that the scapulae become "heavy," and to narrow across the front of the shoulders. This causes the flexors of the arms and the muscles that support the shoulder joint, the rotator cuff, to overwork. It also disorganizes the scapulae muscles so that they don't get the support they need in back. Worst of all, it causes the shoulder girdle to squeeze or collapse downward onto the ribs, impeding the freedom of the ribs and interfering with the natural length and support of the trunk.

In order for the shoulder girdle to work properly, the shoulders must release in the pectoral region, where they tend to become narrowed and where the scapulae become pinned down to the ribs at one of their key attachment points, the coracoid process (Fig. 5-7). In addition to this, the back muscles must widen and fill out so that the scapula can become fully supported within their network of muscles and the rotator cuff muscles around the shoulder joint can release and allow the scapulae to reintegrate into the back.

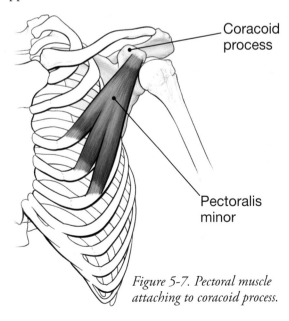

Coracoid process

Pectoralis minor

Figure 5-7. Pectoral muscle attaching to coracoid process.

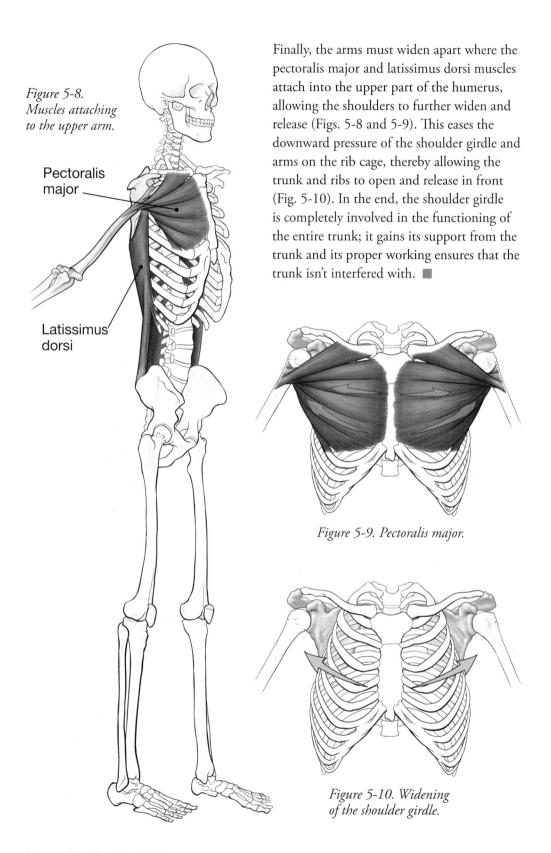

Figure 5-8.
Muscles attaching
to the upper arm.

Pectoralis
major

Latissimus
dorsi

Finally, the arms must widen apart where the pectoralis major and latissimus dorsi muscles attach into the upper part of the humerus, allowing the shoulders to further widen and release (Figs. 5-8 and 5-9). This eases the downward pressure of the shoulder girdle and arms on the rib cage, thereby allowing the trunk and ribs to open and release in front (Fig. 5-10). In the end, the shoulder girdle is completely involved in the functioning of the entire trunk; it gains its support from the trunk and its proper working ensures that the trunk isn't interfered with. ◼

Figure 5-9. Pectoralis major.

Figure 5-10. Widening
of the shoulder girdle.

6. The Upper Limb

In the last two chapters we looked at the shoulder girdle, which functions primarily as a framework for the freely-moving arms. Let's turn now to the design of the arm and hand.

The Basic Limb Pattern

Put simply, the arm is a system of levers that move and position the hand, which in turn is designed for grasping and manipulating objects. The arm is made up of two levers that hinge at the elbow; these levers are quite long so that we can reach and position the hand in a wide arc around the body and in widely varying movements. The upper arm moves very freely at the ball-and-socket joint of the shoulder, which is the most mobile joint in the body. The shoulder, then, is basically a kind of scaffolding that supports the arms, which function as a lever system for moving the hands.

If you look at the bones that make up the upper limb, you'll notice that they follow a pattern quite similar to that of the lower limb: one long bone for the upper arm (the humerus) followed by two bones for the forearm (the ulna and radius). A cluster of wrist, or carpal, bones corresponds to the tarsal bones of the ankle, followed by a series of bones in the hand which are similar in arrangement to those of the foot (Fig. 6-1). In anatomical position (standing with palms facing forward), the ulna is the bone that forms a joint with the humerus at the elbow and goes down the inner side of the forearm in line with the small finger. The radius lies on the thumb side of the forearm. Human arms are proportionately longer than the forelimbs of other animals, since we evolved from apes that needed long limbs for swinging in the trees. At the shoulder, the humerus moves very freely in its shallow "socket"; the elbow joint is a simple hinge that makes it possible to flex and extend the arm in order to reach for and grasp objects.

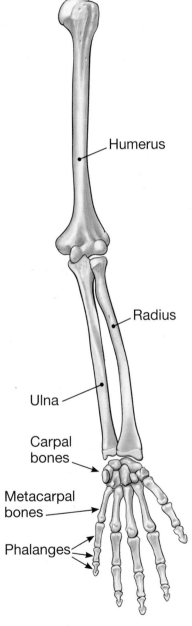

Figure 6-1. Bones of the left upper limb.

Modes of Positioning the Hand

Being able to reach for an object, however, does not mean we will be able to position the hand in such a way that we will be able to grasp the object effectively. The foot of a dog or cat is designed primarily for support and locomotion and moves essentially in one plane; it is simply placed on the ground and pushed off to produce forward movement. The human hand, in contrast, is designed for grasping and manipulating objects; to accomplish this effectively, it must be possible to orient the hand in a variety of ways. The most obvious way we do this is by moving the hand at the wrist, which we can do in two ways. First, we can flex and extend at the wrist (Fig. 6-2b); second, we can deviate the hand sideways (Fig. 6-2a).

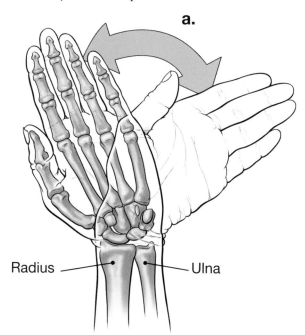

a.

Radius ——— ——— Ulna

Figure 6-2. Action of the hand at the wrist: a. radial and ulnar deviation; b. extension and flexion.

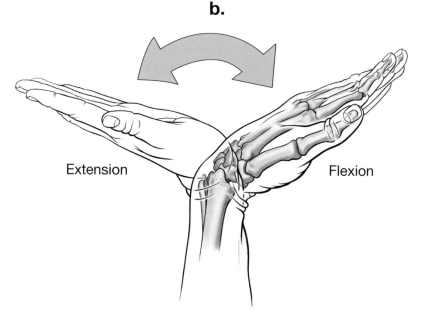

b.

Extension   Flexion

It is also possible to rotate the hand at the forearm. If you raise your left arm at the elbow with the palm facing up, the two bones of the forearm, the radius and ulna, lie parallel. If you turn your hand over, or pronate the forearm, the radius crosses over the ulna, causing the palm to face downward. The reverse motion, or supination, turns the palm upward (Fig. 6-3). The radius, which means "a ray or spoke of a wheel," is given this name because it forms the radius of movement in pronation and supination. Coupled with the movements of the hand at the wrist, movement of the hand at the forearm makes it possible to orient the hand in all three spatial planes, so that it can be positioned quite freely for the purpose of grasping and manipulating things.

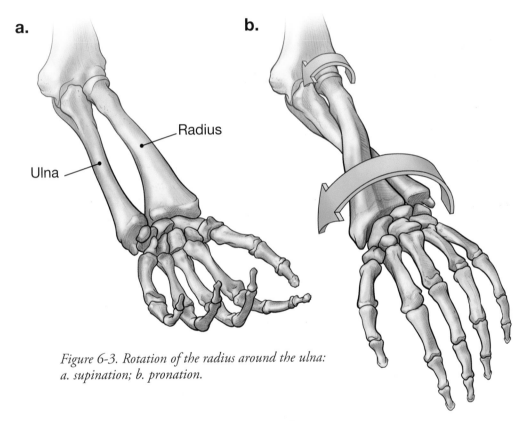

Figure 6-3. Rotation of the radius around the ulna:
a. supination; b. pronation.

The Rotation Mechanism of the Forearm

Let's look at the ingenious design of the wrist and forearm which makes this rotational movement possible. We saw a moment ago that the humerus and ulna form the hinge joint of the elbow and that the radius lies parallel to the ulna. But which bone does the hand articulate with? Many people, when asked this question, point to the ulna, reasoning that since the ulna forms a joint with the elbow, the hand must articulate with the other end of the ulna so that when the ulna moves, the hand moves with it. But the purpose of rotating the radius around the ulna is to pronate the hand so that it can be rotated in relation to the ulna. If the hand were connected to the ulna, or to both the radius and ulna, you wouldn't be able to rotate the hand at all since it would be stuck in a fixed position at the end of the forearm. If, however, the hand were to articulate with the radius and not with the ulna, then it would still be possible to move the hand at the wrist, but with an added advantage: when the radius rotates around the ulna, the hand would go with it—which is precisely the way it works (Fig. 6-4).

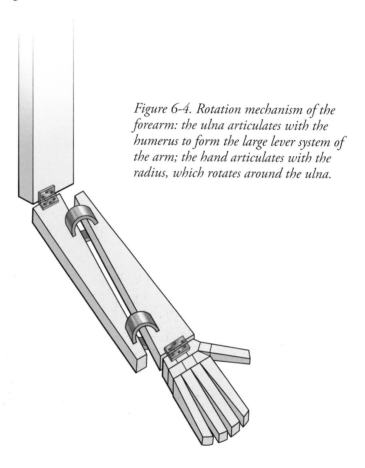

Figure 6-4. Rotation mechanism of the forearm: the ulna articulates with the humerus to form the large lever system of the arm; the hand articulates with the radius, which rotates around the ulna.

To summarize, the humerus and ulna articulate to form the large hinge joint of the elbow, which makes it possible to move the large levers of the arm. But the hand articulates, not with the ulna but with the radius, so that the radius—and the hand with it—can rotate around the ulna. This simple and elegant mechanism makes it possible to pronate and supinate the hand around the ulna while still being able to move the hand freely at the wrist.

The Hand

Let's look now at the hand and the muscles that move it. The hand is made up of five metacarpal bones (which form the palm), and the phalanges which make up the fingers and thumb—two for the thumb and three for each finger (Fig. 6-5). The last two joints of the fingers, the interphalangeal joints, are hinge joints for flexing and extending the fingers. The first joint of the fingers, or knuckle joint, is called the metacarpophalangeal joint because it's formed by the metacarpal bone and the phalange. In addition to being able to flex and extend, it's capable of sideways movement, or adduction and abduction.

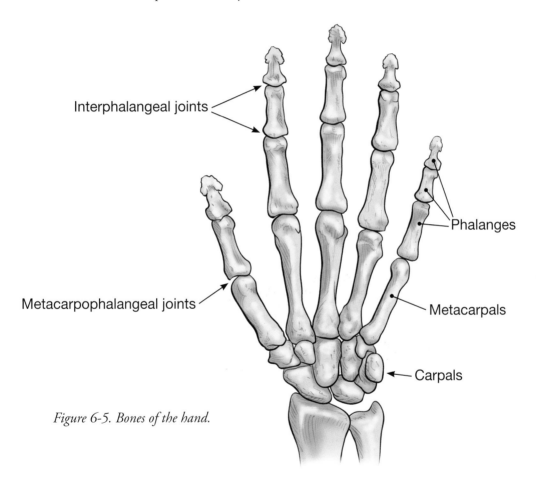

Figure 6-5. Bones of the hand.

The main function of the hand is to grasp things; for this purpose, there are a number of muscles on the palm side of the forearm that powerfully flex the wrist and fingers by means of tendons which pass over the wrist joint and attach to the bones of the wrist and fingers (these are called the "extrinsic" muscles of the hand because they are not part of the hand itself). Because they are located on the forearm, these muscles are able to exert greater power and leverage than the smaller intrinsic muscles of the hand. Extrinsic muscles on the back side of the forearm extend the hand and fingers; because the main purpose of the hand is to flex and grasp things, the flexors are stronger and more numerous than the extensors.

The hand and fingers are also moved by a number of intrinsic muscles—that is, muscles that are part of the hand itself. These include: the muscles that act on the thumb (which form the fleshy pad at the base of the thumb); the muscles of the little finger (which form the pad on that part of the hand); and the muscles of the palm which act on the fingers (and occupy the spaces between the fingers). These muscles make it possible to perform some of the finer movements of the hand—such as opposing the little finger to the other fingers, cupping the palm, splaying the fingers, and opposing the thumb to the fingers.

A particularly interesting group of intrinsic muscles, the lumbricals, flexes the first digits of the fingers while simultaneously extending the second and third digits—that is, it flexes the fingers at the knuckles but keeps them straight from that point. This muscle makes it possible to grasp objects between the thumb and fingers with delicacy and precision and is useful for such activities as holding a pencil or threading a needle (Fig. 6-6).

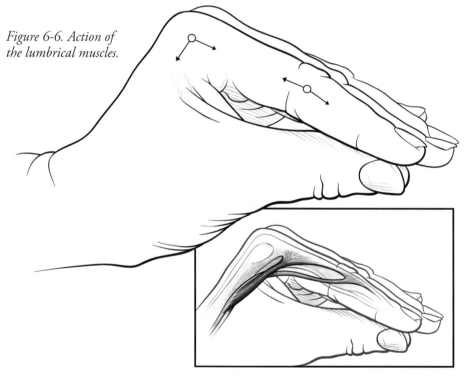

Figure 6-6. Action of the lumbrical muscles.

Inset: tendons of the lumbrical muscles flex the fingers at the metacarpophalangeal joints and extend them at the interphalangeal joints.

The Opposable Thumb

The most versatile and crucial element of the human hand, of course, is the opposable thumb, which makes possible a broad repertoire of prehensile movements—more colloquially known as grasping things. The thumb comprises no fewer than five bones and four joints (Fig. 6-7); its movements are controlled by nine muscles. Four of these muscles are on the forearm (the extrinsic muscles of the thumb); five are on the pad of the thumb (the intrinsic muscles). These muscles make it possible to form a powerful grip, to oppose the thumb to all or each of the fingers, to handle delicate instruments, to grasp tools and weapons, to write, and to form a dynamic grip as in playing a stringed instrument—a remarkable range of skilled activities without which civilization itself would not have been possible.

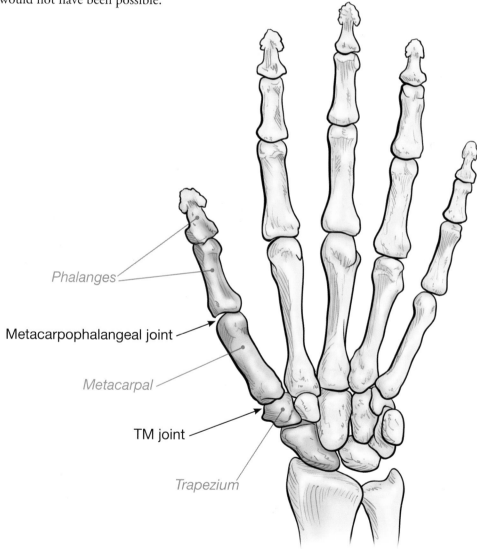

Phalanges

Metacarpophalangeal joint

Metacarpal

TM joint

Trapezium

Figure 6-7. Bones and joints of the thumb.

There are two prominent joints that contribute to the action of the thumb. The outermost or distal joint of the thumb (the one nearest the nail) is basically a hinge, which makes it easier to grip things. The next joint is located at the crook of the thumb and corresponds to the knuckle joints of the fingers. At this joint we can both flex the thumb and move it sideways (Fig. 6-8). Both of these joints are fairly visible and clearly contribute to the thumb's opposing action.

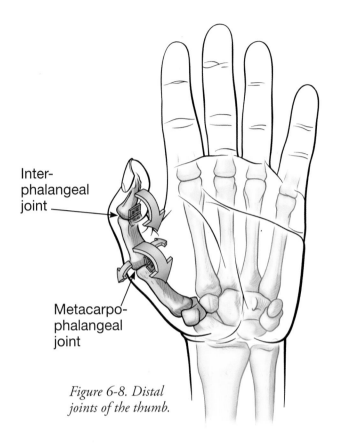

Figure 6-8. Distal joints of the thumb.

The most important movement of the thumb, however, takes place at a crucial but less obvious joint located right at the wrist. If you try to oppose the thumb to the fingers simply by moving at the two joints we've looked at so far, you'll find that it can't be done. It must be possible to move the entire pad of the thumb so that the thumb as a whole can be moved closer to the palm. The only way this can happen is if the thumb moves at the wrist, so that the entire pad of the thumb can be moved in relation to the rest of the hand, bringing the thumb into opposition with the fingers (Fig. 6-9).

This joint at the base of the thumb is the crucial articulation that makes opposition or prehension possible. Because the metacarpal bones are tied together, the fingers begin at the knuckles (Fig. 6-10). In contrast, however, the thumb is formed by a column of bones that begins at the wrist. And because the thumb must move freely in relation to the hand, the pivotal joint in this column of bones is the one formed at its base by the articulation of the wrist and metacarpal bones—the trapezo-metacarpal or TM joint (Fig. 6-10)—which makes it possible to freely move the pad of the thumb to oppose the thumb and fingers (Fig. 6-9b).

The use of the thumb and hand accounts for much of the complexity of the brain and many of the qualities we associate with being human. One of the great advantages of a fully upright posture is that it frees up the hands for manipulative purposes, which in turn

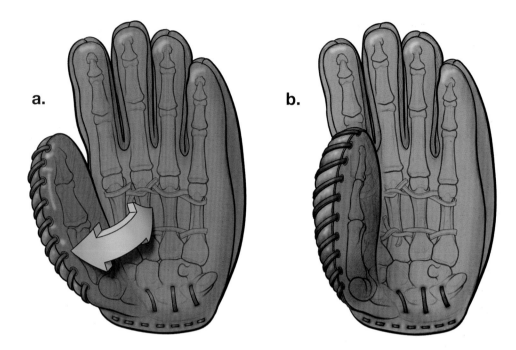

Figure 6-9. Action of TM joint showing how the thumb pad moves in relation to the rest of the hand: a. thumb unopposed to fingers; b. thumb opposed to fingers.

leads to an increased ability to perceive the world three-dimensionally, to build and invent things, to explore the world with our tactile sense, to express ourselves through touch, and to correlate what we see with what we can feel and explore in our environment. This refined use of the hands is largely under our conscious control, so that it becomes a tangible expression of our creative minds.

To summarize, the hand is moved by the long levers of the arm, which move freely from the highly mobile shoulder joint; the hand is positioned by rotation of the forearm and movement at the wrist. The hand itself is capable of very fine and highly controlled movement, including the opposing action of the thumb—a remarkable system that is inextricably linked with our upright design and the evolution of the human brain.

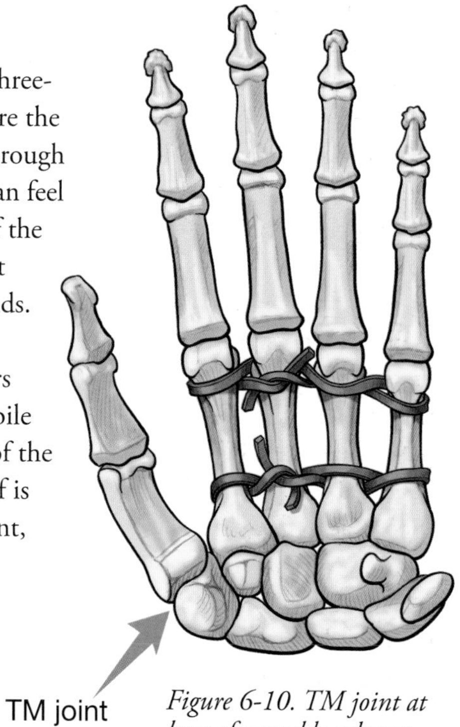

TM joint

Figure 6-10. TM joint at base of movable column.

The Relationship of the Upper Limb to the Shoulder and Trunk

When observed from a purely mechanical point of view, the use of the hand and arm seems for all intents and purposes to be separate from that of the shoulder. But the functioning of the arms is quite dependent on the shoulder girdle, which in turn is dependent on the support system of the trunk. As we saw in the last chapter, a common tendency, in using the arms, is to narrow the shoulders and to overuse the flexors of the arms and fingers. This pattern is intrinsically associated with the tendency to shorten or collapse in front. When we are able to maintain length in the trunk and to keep the shoulders widening while using the arms, then the use of the arms is coordinated with the muscles of the back, the flexors do not over-contract, and the arm and hand function to best advantage. Ultimately, the functioning of the arm and hand is dependent on the muscles supporting the trunk and shoulder girdle and is an integral part of our upright design. ∎

7. The Pelvic Girdle

In Chapter Five, we examined the design of the shoulder girdle. As we discovered, it provides a powerful yet mobile framework for the upper limb, which with upright posture has become mainly manipulative in function. In contrast, the pelvic girdle is designed to provide support on two legs, and has therefore developed quite differently than its upper torso counterpart.

The Design of the Pelvis

The pelvic girdle is basically a bony structure at the bottom end of the spine that provides deep and stable sockets for the hip joints so that we can stand on our own two legs. This ring-like girdle also provides a sturdy framework for muscular attachments to the trunk and legs. Because we are upright, the pelvis also forms a container at the bottom end of the trunk for our innards ("*pelvis*" is a Latin word meaning "basin").

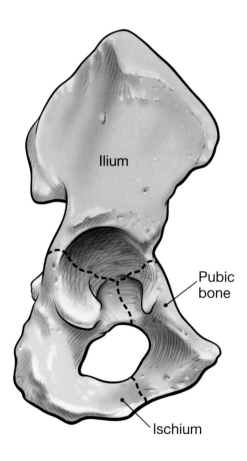

The pelvis is made up of three bones—the ilium, or hip bone; the ischium, which forms the sit bones; and the pubic bone (Fig. 7-1). Unlike the scapula of the shoulder, which is a single bone, the three bones that make up the pelvis became fused together during evolution to form the "scapula" of the pelvic girdle. This is somewhat confusing because, although these bones function as one unit, we still designate parts of the pelvis in terms of these specific bones, such as the iliac crest or the pubic bone. Also, these three bones then become attached to the spine and to each other in front, so that the pelvic bones, the sacral region of the spine, and the pelvis as a whole tend to get confused. All this becomes clearer if you think of the pelvis as consisting of two wing-like structures which, like the scapulae of the shoulder, provide sockets for the limbs but which happen to be made up of three bones each.

Figure 7-1. Bones of the pelvis.

The pelvis, as we can see when we look at a skeleton, has quite an unusual and complex design. First, the two wing-like pelvic bones are firmly attached to either side of the spine. Second, these bones are attached in front to form a ring, or circular girdle. Finally, there are two curved "rockers" at the bottom of the pelvis (the sit bones), forming a complex three-dimensional structure (Fig. 7-2). The Greeks and Romans tended to name anatomical structures according to what they resembled; because the bones making up each side of the pelvis didn't resemble anything, the Romans named it the "innominate bone"—the "bone without a name"!

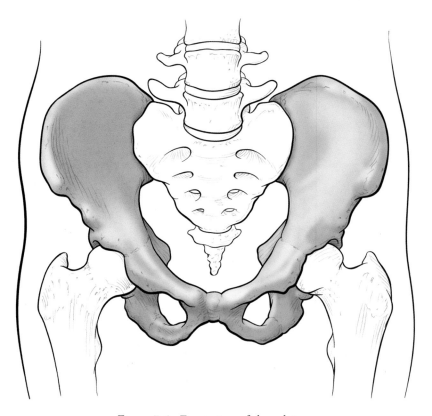

Figure 7-2. Front view of the pelvis.

However, if you consider what the pelvis actually does, it becomes much easier to understand its design. Like the scapula of the shoulder, the pelvis provides bony sockets for the two lower limbs, which originated as fins in fish (Fig. 7-3a). However, the rear legs of a four-footed animal, unlike the front legs, have the job of propelling the animal forward on land. For this reason, the pelvic bones needed to attach directly to the spine so that force from the hind legs could be directly transmitted to the trunk—a crucial design element that's present in all animals that move on the ground (Fig. 7-3b).

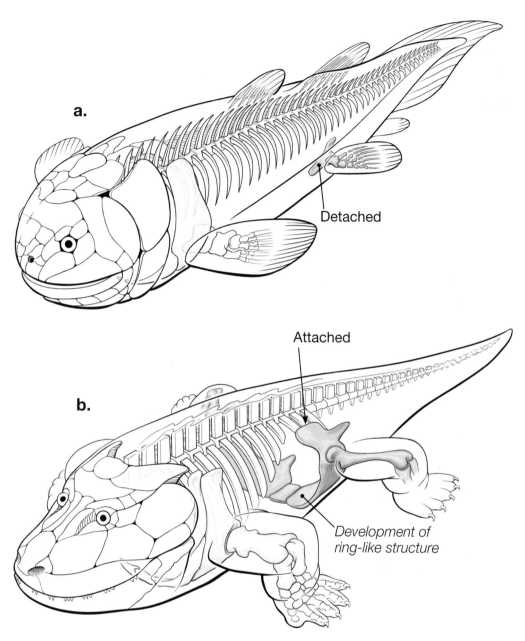

a.

Detached

Attached

b.

Development of
ring-like structure

*Figure 7-3. Relationship of the "scapula" of the pelvis to the spine in:
a. fish (crossopterygian); b. amphibian (labyrinthodont).*

In amphibians and reptiles the legs are splayed out to the sides; in quadrupeds the legs are brought underneath the body so that force from the legs can be more directly transmitted to the spine.

You can see how effective this is in dogs, cats, and hoofed animals when they run, with powerful thrusts of the legs efficiently propelling the body forward (Fig. 7-4a). The forelimbs of a four-footed animal, in contrast, are less involved in propelling the animal forward than in cushioning the body's impact on the ground; this explains why the scapulae of four-footed animals are not attached to the spine but move independently of it (Fig. 7-4b).

The connection of the pelvis with the legs then, provides a means of directly translating movement of the legs into movement of the trunk. This also explains why movement of the pelvis, in contrast to the independent action of the scapula of the shoulder, directly involves movement of the spine. Any movement of the pelvis has to involve the spine because the two are firmly attached. And you can't really speak of the pelvis, as we shall soon learn, without also speaking about the back, since the pelvis functions in many ways as an extension of the back.

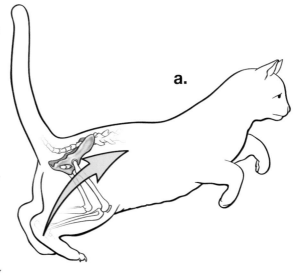

Figure 7-4a. "Scapula" of pelvis is directly connected to spine to transmit force from legs to spine and to support weight of body on legs.

This connection of the pelvis with the spine is marked by one other crucial development. If the pelvic bones of a four-footed animal were attached only at the sacrum, they would not be stable enough for weight-bearing. Animals on land needed a firmer structure so that the pelvis could absorb force from the legs and bear weight without placing undue strain on the sacroiliac joints where the pelvic bones attach to the spine. For this reason, the pubic bones grew forward and around and joined up in front to form a bony ring. Instead of having two blades connected to either side of the spine, the two pelvic bones now formed a solid, ring-like girdle that provided a sturdy framework for the sockets of the femurs and for support and locomotion on four feet (Fig. 7-3b).

The Upright Compromise

If the shoulder and pelvic girdles differ in four-legged animals, the differences become even more pronounced in humans. In our upright posture, the spine and trunk are balanced vertically on the legs, freeing the arms from having to support the body. The upper limb thus becomes mainly manipulative and the shoulder girdle, which now sits on top of the rib cage, becomes quite light and mobile to permit the arms a wide range of movement. The pelvis, meanwhile, not only bears weight; it bears the entire weight of the trunk, which now rests solely on the legs—a tremendous increase in responsibility. For this purpose, the pelvic bones had to become heavier and stronger, and even more firmly fastened onto the sacral part of the spine (which became virtually vestigial from here downwards, so that the tail was dispensed with). In contrast to the shallow and mobile joints of the shoulder, the sockets for the femurs became deeper, providing very stable joints for the femurs.

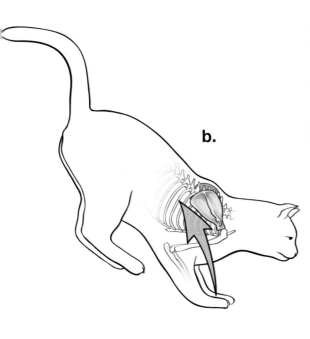

b.

Figure 7-4b. Scapula of the shoulder girdle is unattached in order for force to be absorbed in landing.

The structure now became beautifully suited to carry the entire weight of the trunk on the two hind limbs, thus providing a very solid framework for propulsion and support on two legs. In contrast to the shoulder joint, which sacrificed stability for mobility, the pelvic or hip joint sacrificed mobility for stability. The shoulder is held in place largely by muscles and tendons, but the pelvis has powerful ligaments attaching it to the spine and securing the hip joint, which is very stable and snug. (These ligaments temporarily loosen up during pregnancy in order to make room for the infant's head in childbirth.) This limits the mobility of the hip joint; but it is interesting to consider that this diminished range of motion is compensated for in part by the angle of the femur, which serves to increase the range of motion of the leg at the hip and also provides attachments for the hip muscles that support the hip joint and act on the femur.

The Arch Design of the Pelvis

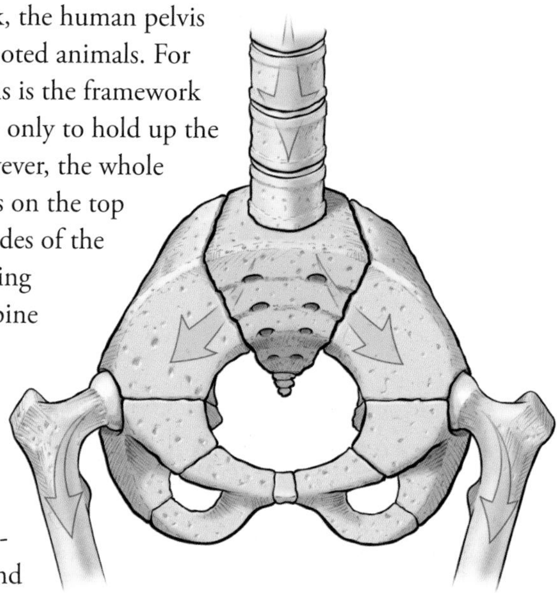

In supporting the vertically-poised trunk, the human pelvis functions differently than that of four-footed animals. For an animal walking on four feet, the pelvis is the framework for supporting the hind legs, which have only to hold up the back end of the animal. In humans, however, the whole of the vertically-poised trunk literally sits on the top ends, or heads, of the femurs. The two sides of the pelvis now become an arch for transmitting weight from the central column of the spine down onto the femurs and into the legs (Fig. 7-5). With the pubic bones joined in front and yet cushioned by a disc much like the intervertebral discs of the spine, this arch design provides a strong and efficient structure for support-ing the weight of the body on two legs and absorbing shock through the circumference of the pelvis when one walks, runs, or jumps.

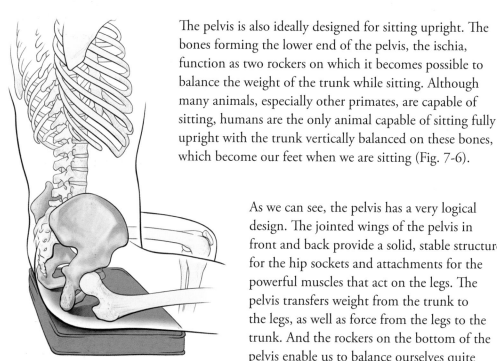

Figure 7-5. Arch of pelvis transmitting weight to legs.

The pelvis is also ideally designed for sitting upright. The bones forming the lower end of the pelvis, the ischia, function as two rockers on which it becomes possible to balance the weight of the trunk while sitting. Although many animals, especially other primates, are capable of sitting, humans are the only animal capable of sitting fully upright with the trunk vertically balanced on these bones, which become our feet when we are sitting (Fig. 7-6).

As we can see, the pelvis has a very logical design. The jointed wings of the pelvis in front and back provide a solid, stable structure for the hip sockets and attachments for the powerful muscles that act on the legs. The pelvis transfers weight from the trunk to the legs, as well as force from the legs to the trunk. And the rockers on the bottom of the pelvis enable us to balance ourselves quite effortlessly in a chair when using our arms in a fully upright sitting posture.

Figure 7-6. The ischial tuberosities form rockers for sitting.

The Pelvis in Relation to Lengthening in Stature

Let's look now at the kinds of muscular support that the pelvis requires. The primary function of the pelvis is to provide sockets for the femurs for support and propulsion on two legs. But few people have a clear idea of the relationship of the legs to the pelvis. When asked where the hip joints are located, many people will point to the hip bones—a misconception which is echoed in the linguistic similarity between the names we use for two very different parts of the pelvis ("hips" versus "hip joints"). In practical terms, this misconception translates into the tendency, when bending or sitting, to make a joint at the waist, which causes the trunk to shorten. To maintain the proper length of the trunk when bending, we must appreciate that for all intents and purposes the pelvis functions as part of the back, and that bending properly takes place, not at the waist, but at the hip joints. Maintaining the full length of the trunk therefore requires that we know where the hip joints are located and how to use them properly.

There is a corollary to this principle of understanding where the hip joints are located. If the pelvis is connected to the spine, and if bending takes place at the hip joints, then the back of the pelvis, or sacral region of the spine, functions not as part of the legs but as part of the length of the back. In Chapter Two we saw that the sacrospinalis muscles extend from the sacrum right up to the base of the skull; in anatomical terms, the sacral region provides a stable point of origin for the extensor muscles running up the length of the back. This means that the pelvis is more than a stable support structure for the legs and its muscular attachments; it is in fact part of the back and must be thought of this way if we are to maintain a fully lengthened trunk.

The connection between the pelvis and the spine is made even more intimate by the fact that, to achieve a fully upright posture, the human spine had to develop a lumbar curve (see Figs. 4-5 and 4-7), which creates instability in the lower back. The iliopsoas muscle, which crosses the inside of the pelvis as it passes from the lumbar spine to the femur, plays a crucial role in stabilizing the pelvis in relation to the back (Fig. 7-7).

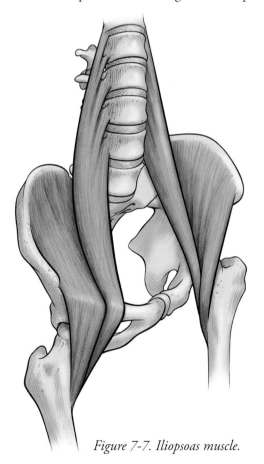

Figure 7-7. Iliopsoas muscle.

In conjunction with the erector spinae muscles, it maintains the support and length of the lower back (Fig. 7-8). When we slump and collapse the spine, however, the back muscles become contracted and the iliopsoas muscle, which also becomes shortened, pulls on the lower back. In order to restore natural length and support in the trunk, the iliopsoas muscle must release across the front of the pelvis. Roughly corresponding to the freeing of the pectoral region of the chest which allows the

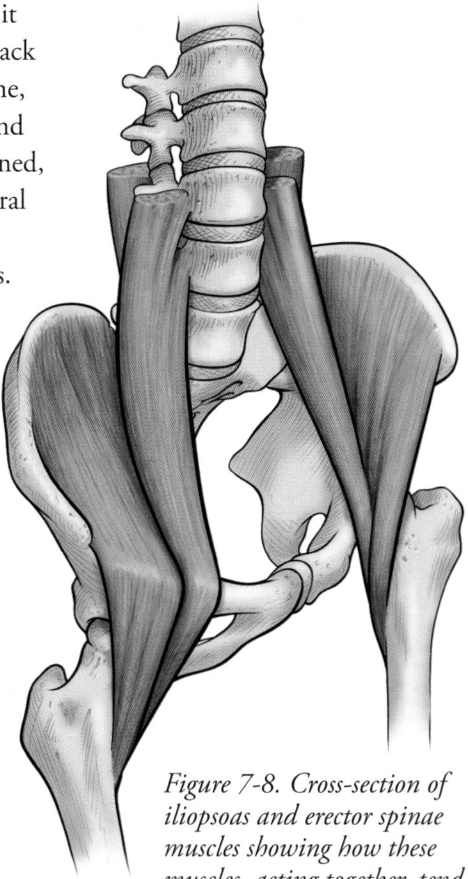

Figure 7-8. Cross-section of iliopsoas and erector spinae muscles showing how these muscles, acting together, tend to straighten and support the lumbar curve of the spine.

shoulder girdle to widen, this frontal release of the iliopsoas muscle allows the lower back to lengthen and the thighs to release out of the hips, and is thus a crucial element in restoring the lengthened support of the trunk (Fig. 7-9). In this sense, the fate of the lower back is completely intertwined with the pelvis and its connection with the trunk. To coordinate properly, the legs must integrate with the lower back in such a way that they don't pull the pelvis and lower back out of balance or cause shortening in the iliopsoas muscles that support this region. ■

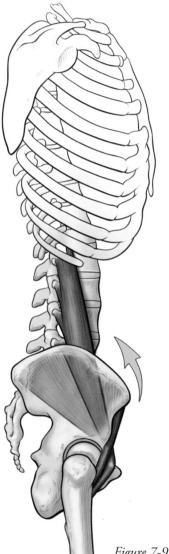

Figure 7-9. Side view of the spine and pelvis showing the release of the psoas muscle in supporting the pelvis.

8. The Lower Limb

In the last chapter, we looked at the upper limb and how its design makes it possible to grasp and manipulate objects. In contrast, the lower limb is of course designed for support on two feet. For this purpose, it is much stronger than the arm; it carries weight directly above the ground by means of bones which are stacked on top of one another and ultimately rest on the arched foot; and it has quite powerful muscles for propulsion and support. Let's take a closer look at the unique design features of the lower limb.

The Weight-Bearing Limb

The leg, like the arm, is basically a system of levers, except that the leg has retained its original function of support and locomotion. For this reason, the leg bones are long and strong, the hip joint is deep and stable, the knee joint is large, the leg muscles are powerful and plentiful (there are nearly twice as many muscles in the leg as in the arm), and the foot is no longer prehensile (as it is in our ape relatives) but has become a shock absorber. Yet, in spite of the fact that we carry our weight on the legs and move them in fairly circumscribed ways compared to the arm, the leg and foot are nevertheless capable of a complex range of movement—in particular, at the hip, the ankle, and the foot, which is constantly being adjusted to the ground by the muscles of the lower leg.

Like the upper limb, the leg is comprised of one long bone (the femur), followed by two lower leg bones (the tibia and fibula), a cluster of tarsal, or ankle bones, and the bones of the foot (the metatarsals and phalanges)—three for each little toe and two for the big toe (Fig. 8-1). As with the upper limb, the long bone of the leg forms a ball-and-socket joint with its supporting girdle. The long bones of the leg hinge at the knee, and the foot can be moved and adjusted in relation to the lower leg, not for the purpose of grasping objects (the big toe has lost the ability to oppose the other toes), but in order to adjust the foot to the ground for balance and movement.

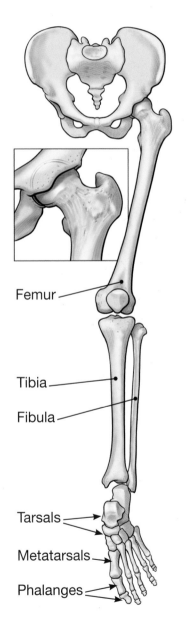

Figure 8-1. Bones of the lower limb.

The most obvious function of the leg is to support the body off the ground and to move it in space. Obviously the bones alone can't do this; it takes muscles to move and stabilize them. The main muscles of the legs are the extensors on the front of the thigh, which as we saw are part of the larger extensor system that supports us against gravity (see Fig. 2-1 on page 7); the flexors or hamstrings on the back of the thigh; and the adductors on the inside of the thigh. When we brace and tighten the legs, we shorten these muscles, which then need to release so that the legs regain their spring and elasticity.

In the last chapter, we saw how the pelvis serves as an arch to transmit the weight of the trunk onto the heads of the femurs. This weight is carried from the femur onto the tibia, the large bone of the lower leg, which sits on the talus and the heel bone (Fig. 8-2). Notice that the weight from the femur sits entirely on the tibia, which in turn sits on the talus and the arch of the foot; the fibula does not bear any weight at all (see Fig. 8-3). This means that we have a direct bony connection from the feet right up through the tibia, femur, pelvis, spine, and on up to the skull, which is perched on top of the whole structure.

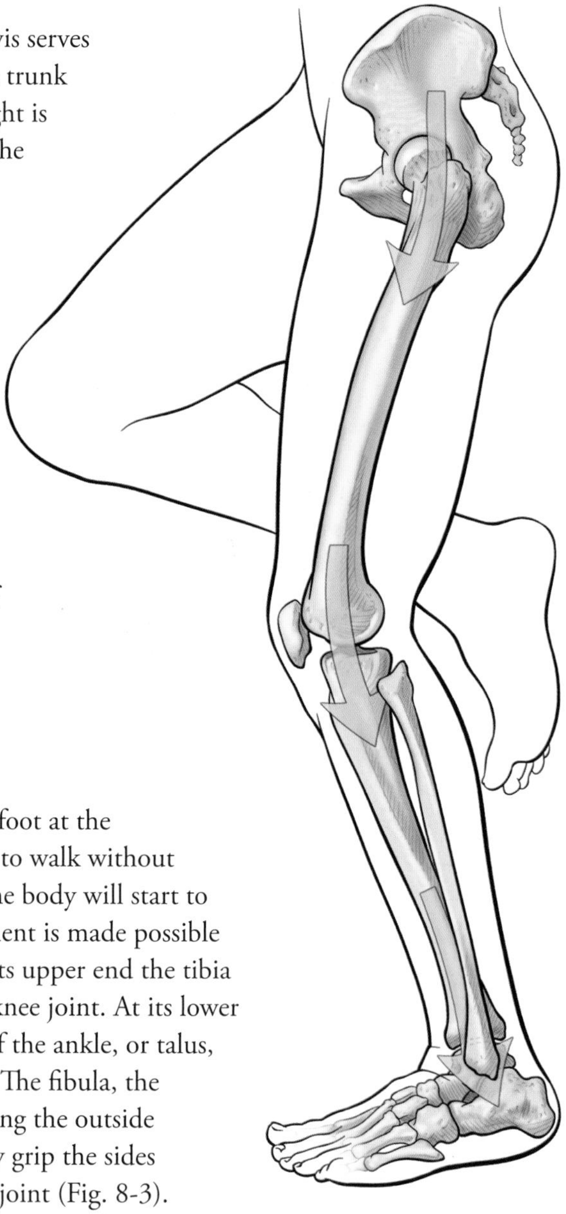

The Ankle Joint

Let's look now at the movement of the foot at the ankle. If you stand normally and begin to walk without actually taking a step, you'll find that the body will start to pivot forward at the ankle. This movement is made possible by the ankle joint. We just saw that at its upper end the tibia articulates with the femur to form the knee joint. At its lower end, the tibia sits on the central bone of the ankle, or talus, and also wraps around it on the inside. The fibula, the other bone of the lower leg, extends along the outside of the talus so that the two bones firmly grip the sides of the talus to form a stable, hinge-like joint (Fig. 8-3). The talus is able to move within these bones (called the malleoli), allowing dorsiflexion and plantar flexion of the

Figure 8-2. Distribution of weight on the leg bones.

foot—that is, bringing the toes toward the shin, and extending the foot away from the shin (Fig. 8-4).

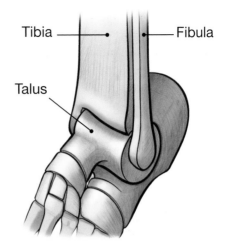

Notice how this joint differs from the wrist. Whereas only one bone of the forearm articulates with the wrist, both bones of the lower leg participate in the ankle joint. This is because the ankle, which bears weight, requires greater stability than the wrist joint. So the bottom end of the tibia sits on top of and articulates with the talus, which is the central ankle bone. At their lower ends, the malleoli of the tibia and fibula grip the talus on the sides like a pincer, forming a hinge joint. If you flex the ankle while

Figure 8-3. The ankle joint.

pinching these two bones between your fingers, you will feel the movement of the talus directly in between these "pincers." You can also feel the upper end of the fibula move as it accommodates to the movement of the talus within the tibia and fibula.

The fibula serves another very important function. Obviously the lower leg needs to be strong enough to withstand the stresses of running, leaping, and jumping. Bone, however, is heavy, and humans require fairly light bones in order to move easily, unlike larger and heavier animals that are less

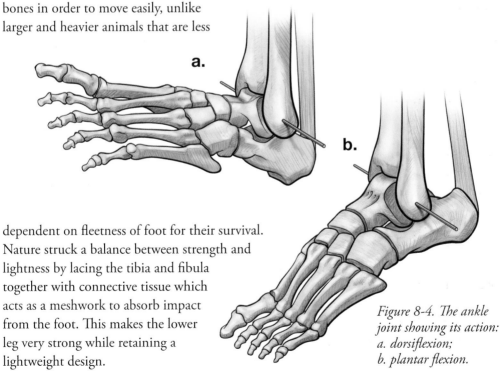

dependent on fleetness of foot for their survival. Nature struck a balance between strength and lightness by lacing the tibia and fibula together with connective tissue which acts as a meshwork to absorb impact from the foot. This makes the lower leg very strong while retaining a lightweight design.

Figure 8-4. The ankle joint showing its action: a. dorsiflexion; b. plantar flexion.

The Foot Joints

The ankle joint, however, is not the only important joint allowing movement of the foot. If you move your foot at the ankle you'll find that it is possible, not simply to hinge at the ankle, but to rotate the foot freely as if the ankle is a ball-and-socket joint. As we've seen, however, the talus, which is the keystone of the foot, is firmly held within the pincers of the malleoli and can only hinge at this point. The sideways movements of the foot occur not at the ankle joint, where the talus hinges with the tibia and fibula of the lower leg, but where the front of the foot and heel bone articulate with the talus. These joints, which are technically not ankle but foot joints, enable the foot to orient itself sideways with respect to the ground—that is, to flex and turn face in (inversion), or to extend and turn face out (eversion) (Fig. 8-5). These movements are crucial because if you could only hinge the foot at the ankle, the foot would not be able to maintain its contact with the ground when confronted with unevenness in terrain or changes in the position of the leg (as when pushing off on one foot).

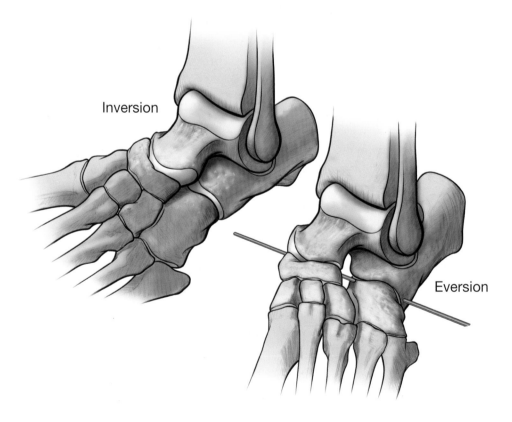

Figure 8-5. Transverse joint showing its action: inversion and eversion of the foot.

The Arched Foot

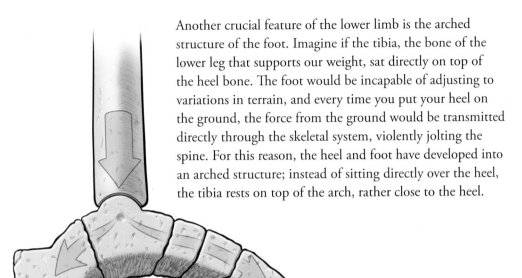

Another crucial feature of the lower limb is the arched structure of the foot. Imagine if the tibia, the bone of the lower leg that supports our weight, sat directly on top of the heel bone. The foot would be incapable of adjusting to variations in terrain, and every time you put your heel on the ground, the force from the ground would be transmitted directly through the skeletal system, violently jolting the spine. For this reason, the heel and foot have developed into an arched structure; instead of sitting directly over the heel, the tibia rests on top of the arch, rather close to the heel.

Figure 8-6. Where the lower leg sits on the arch of the foot.

Weight from the tibia is therefore partly distributed forward into the foot, and the arch of the foot, which is really made up of movable joints and is therefore able to flexibly adapt to pressure and variability in terrain, can absorb shock from the ground (Fig. 8-6). This arched design also gives the foot several points of support so that we can better balance on two feet.

The arches of the foot have a simple and elegant architectural structure. Most people think of the foot as having one long arch running between the big toe and the heel. But the foot actually has three points of support for bearing weight—the ball of the big toe, the ball of the little toe, and the heel, with arches between each of them—forming a kind of three-sided vaulted structure, or "plantar vault," as it's sometimes called (Fig. 8-7).

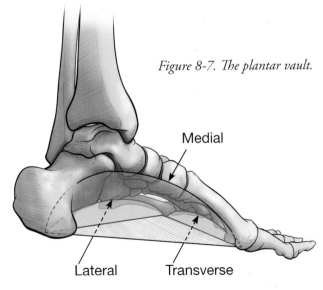

Figure 8-7. The plantar vault.

Medial

Lateral

Transverse

The main arch is called the "medial arch"; it is easy to feel along the inside of the foot and clearly comes up off the ground (Fig. 8-8a). The arch between the ball of the little toe and heel runs along the outside of the foot and is called the "lateral arch" (Fig. 8-8b); it isn't so easy to feel because it is filled by muscle. Finally, the arch across the front of the foot is called the transverse arch, which is also difficult to feel (Fig. 8-8c).

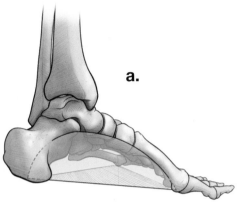

a.

The arches are easy to identify if you pinpoint the three main weight bearing areas—the ball of the big toe, the ball of the little toe, and the heel—and draw lines between them, forming a triangle. The three lines of the triangle describe the three arches—two longitudinal arches (along the length of the foot) and one transverse arch (along the width of the foot)—which act as an elastic shock absorber and permit the foot to adjust to uneven terrain (Fig. 8-9).

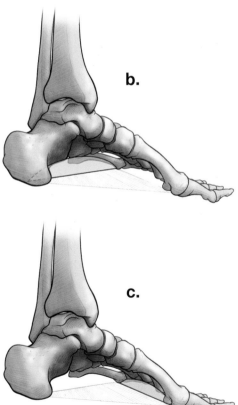

b.

c.

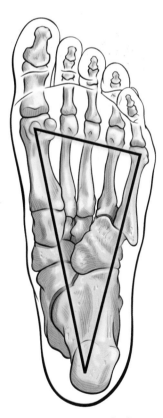

Figure 8-8. The arches: a. medial arch; b. lateral arch; c. transverse arch.

Figure 8-9. Triangle showing the three arches of the foot.

The Toes

The toe joints resemble those of the hand but are specifically adapted for bearing weight and walking. As with the fingers and thumb, there are three joints in each toe and two in the big toe; they are all hinge joints except for the metatarsal joints, which are also capable, just like the knuckle joints of the fingers, of adduction and abduction. The toes, however, differ from the fingers in two fundamental respects. First, the fingers are rather long, are designed to flex in order to grasp objects, and do not extend a great deal; the toes, in contrast, have become much shorter and are therefore no longer very efficient for grasping objects or opposing the big toe, and can bend backwards in order to accommodate to the ground during walking. Second, the big toe has lost the ability to oppose the other digits. The main joint of the big toe, the metatarsophalangeal joint, is particularly important for balance and propulsion because it allows the ball of the foot to be actively pushed off as the leg is advanced. The other joints of the toes are used only minimally to aid in balance.

Length in the Legs

We've observed that in the upright posture, there's a common tendency to pull back the head, to shorten the back muscles, and to collapse and shorten in front. This is usually accompanied by a corresponding tendency to pull the hips forward and sink into the legs. When this happens, the legs become stiffened and braced at the knees, and the muscles of the inner thigh become chronically contracted. In order to restore length and proper support to the system, not only must we activate the muscles of the trunk, but we must also restore the lengthened support of the muscles of the buttocks, the inner thigh, and the backs of the leg (Fig. 8-10). This in turn takes pressure off the hip joints and helps the legs to regain their springiness.

Shortening in the legs is also connected with a loss of mobility in the foot and ankle joints—a tendency that is often pronounced in elderly people, who shuffle their feet when they walk because the ankle will not bend. When we shorten in stature and brace our legs, the foot and ankle also become braced; the challenge then becomes to restore the natural length of the leg muscles and the mobility of the ankle and foot joints, whose movements are part and parcel of our upright design.

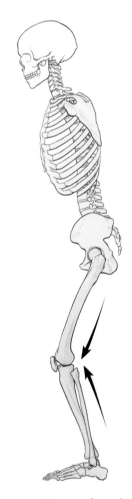

Figure 8-10. Length in the legs.

Our Two-Footed Poise

Although other animals are able to walk on two feet, only humans are capable of a fully upright, striding gait. Walking is initiated when the body, which pivots at the ankles, inclines forward; by allowing one of the knees to bend, the leg swings forward at the hip and straightens as it comes underneath the body so that the trunk is now supported by the advanced leg. By alternately allowing each leg to swing underneath the trunk as the body moves forward, we stride forward effortlessly, exhibiting a fully upright means of locomotion that is unique in the animal kingdom.

Because humans have evolved as bipeds, the body is unstably poised at the ankle joint and is able to move forward because of this instability. The design of the foot is directly related to this instability. A four-footed animal is stable both sideways and front-to-back; but on two feet, we lose our front-to-back stability and can easily topple forward, as we can see when a young child is learning to walk. The length of the human foot and its three points of support, as well as the muscles of the foot, ankle, and lower leg, compensate for this instability, giving us the ability to adjust our foot and lower leg in relation to the ground and to maintain our balance when standing.

To summarize, the weight of the tibia, and indeed the entire body, sits on top of the arched foot like a vaulted bridge, and the bones which make up this bridge are movable so that the entire foot can flexibly adapt to the pressure from above and changes in the terrain from below. At the same time, the foot, including the arch, is supported by ligaments and muscles that register subtle changes in mechanical pressure and help to stabilize the legs and feet. Textbooks on movement often describe the muscles of the legs and feet in terms of the specific actions they make, as when you flex a toe or invert the foot. But these muscles evolved mainly in the context of balance and propulsion on two feet, as well as prehension and swinging in the trees—a remarkable structure beautifully adapted for balance and movement on two feet.

This anatomical design, in turn, is directly related to the evolution of our higher faculties. In previous chapters we saw that the head balances on top of the spine and that the pelvis, which is connected to the spine, balances on top of the heads of the femurs. As we've seen in this chapter, the femurs in turn balance on the tibia at the knee and the tibia sits on top of the talus and the arch of the foot. This balancing act is what made the human striding gait possible, completely freed the arms so that the hands could be used for tool-making, and led ultimately to the development of the human brain. Civilization, science, the arts, writing, religion—all are ultimately made possible by the wonderful balancing act of our physical anatomical design. ■

9. Breathing

In the last chapter we looked at the lower limb, which is designed for balance and locomotion on two feet, and contrasted it with the upper limb, which is designed for grasping and manipulating objects. Along with the head and trunk, these systems comprise the most obvious structures in the body relating to movement. Let's take a look now at two crucial systems, the vocal mechanism and breathing, that tend to be neglected in discussions of functional anatomy and movement. We'll begin with the most basic of these: breathing.

Why and How We Breathe

Breathing is a vital life function. All day long, every day of our lives, we must take in air to provide cells throughout our body with oxygen. Unlike many basic life functions, however, breathing is not a process that only occurs "internally," like kidney function or peristalsis, but is directly linked with the ongoing activity of our musculoskeletal system, for the simple reason that breathing involves an exchange of gases, and this exchange takes place by increasing and decreasing the space within our rib cage—in other words, through movement. When we increase this space, air rushes into our lungs; when we decrease it, air is forced out. This inflow and outflow of air is what we call breathing.

But exactly how do we increase and decrease the space within our bodies? We do it in two ways. First, the ribs rise like pail handles, which expands the overall size of the rib cage (Fig. 9-1).

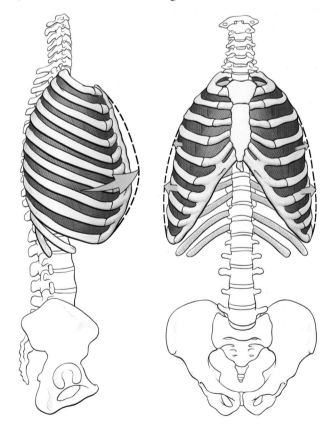

Figure 9-1. Movement of the ribs during inhalation and exhalation.

Second, the diaphragm, which is a dome-shaped muscle that forms the lower boundary of the thorax, flattens out and thus creates more space in the lower part of the thorax (Figs. 9-2 and 9-3). If these two movements are interfered with through muscular tension and collapse, then breathing will not take place efficiently and the diaphragm will have to work harder to ensure that enough air comes into the lungs. Ideally, however, breathing should occur easily and naturally, as a result of the coordinated working of the entire musculature.

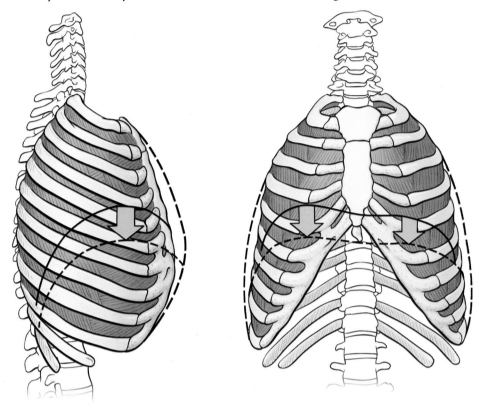

Figure 9-2. Movement of the diaphragm during inhalation and exhalation.

The Anatomy of Breathing

We are all familiar with the basic design of the rib cage (Fig. 9-4). There are twelve ribs on each side of the body, corresponding to the twelve thoracic vertebrae of the spine. The first seven ribs attach in front to the sternum, or breastbone; these are called true ribs. The remaining five join each other to form an arch below the sternum called the "costal arch"; these are called "false ribs" because they don't attach directly to the sternum. The final two ribs are called "floating ribs" because they don't go all the way around to join in front and therefore "float" freely. Interestingly, the ribs are not bony all the way around. Before reaching the sternum they become cartilage, so that the connection of the ribs with the sternum, as well as the costal arch, is cartilaginous and quite flexible.

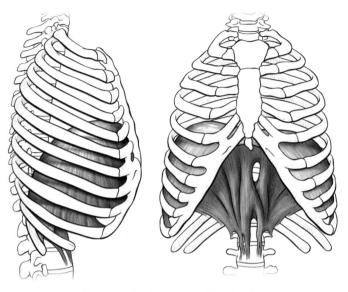

The rib cage is a critical component of our upright support system. We saw earlier that the extensor muscles run up the back and work with the spine to support us in the upright posture. These muscles attach not only to the spine but also to the ribs, which act as struts, or attachment points, for the muscles of the back, as well as for the muscles that wrap around the trunk and abdomen.

Figure 9-3. Anatomy of the diaphragm.

A primary function of the rib cage, of course, is to provide space and protection for the heart and lungs. The heart sits right behind the lower part of the sternum and a little to the left; the lungs are on either side of the heart.

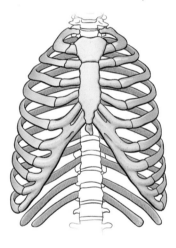

Figure 9-4. Anatomy of the rib cage.

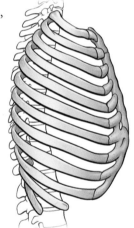

The diaphragm constitutes the lower boundary of the thorax; the heart and lungs lie above the diaphragm, and all the other major internal organs lie below the diaphragm, which forms a boundary between these upper and lower regions of the trunk (Fig. 9-5). The word "diaphragm" is actually a descriptive term that the Greeks gave to this muscle: it means "partition wall."

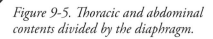

Figure 9-5. Thoracic and abdominal contents divided by the diaphragm.

We normally do not think of the ribs as possessing joints, but it's the movement of the ribs in relation to the spine that produces breathing. When we breathe in, the ribs rotate like pail handles being raised slightly. The raising of the ribs increases the lateral dimension of the thorax, and the raising of the sternum in front increases the antero-posterior dimensions of the thorax as well (Fig. 9-1). At the same time, the diaphragm contracts and flattens out (Fig. 9-2). The combined movements of the ribs and diaphragm increase the space within the thorax, and air rushes into our lungs. When the ribs descend and the diaphragm goes back up, the space in the thorax is decreased, and air is forced out of the lungs.

Notice that air enters the lungs entirely as a result of the fact that we increase the space inside the thorax, not because we've actively drawn it in through our nose or mouth. In this sense, breathing, or the exchange of air, is the passive result of bodily movements and depends entirely on the quality of these movements to work efficiently.

The Suspensory Support of the Trunk

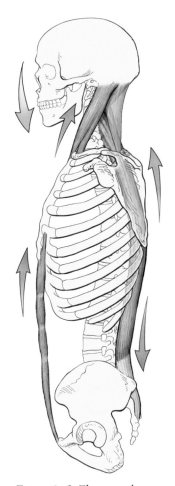

What happens in many of us, however, is that we interfere with this freedom of movement by tensing and collapsing the body and distorting the shape of the thorax. As we saw in Chapters Two and Three, the trunk is supported by the extensors in back and the flexors in front, and the ribs are literally suspended from above by muscles, so that the openness and freedom of the rib cage is dependent on the proper length and support of the entire trunk (Fig. 9-6). In four-footed animals, the ribs hang from the spine, which functions as a kind of bridge that supports the ribs between the fore and hind limbs. In humans, however, the spine is vertical and the ribs, although sloping downward, extend forwards and must therefore be suspended from above. The human ribs thus depend on the vertical support system for support and mobility. When the spine and trunk are properly lengthening, the rib cage will be open and the ribs will be able to move freely. If we lose this support, however, the entire trunk becomes distorted and the ribs in turn become rigid. The rib cage as a whole becomes fixed in the wrong attitude, forcing the diaphragm, the other main agent of breathing, to overwork to make up for the diminished mobility of the ribs.

Figure 9-6. Flexor and extensor support of the rib cage.

When the trunk is properly supported and the back is naturally lengthening, this tends to reorient the rib cage, allowing the upper chest and rib cage to open up and increasing the mobility and freedom of the ribs. In this sense, bringing length to the system restores widening to the ribs. Put simply, the proper condition of the thorax and freedom of movement of the ribs and, therefore, the breathing function as well, depend on the lengthening of this system against gravity. Our breathing function is integrally related to our unique upright design.

There is another sense in which lengthening brings about widening and freeing of the ribs. We've seen that the long extensor muscles of the back act in concert with the spine to maintain erect posture. When the back is shortened and narrowed, some of these extensors become flaccid and lose muscle tone; others are chronically contracted and pin the ribs down by tugging on them from below. When the back lengthens and the head is balancing forward and going up, the extensor muscles release and allow the ribs to expand. Lengthening the back, in other words, allows the ribs to expand; once again, lengthening brings about widening.

Widening the Back

But what exactly does it mean for the back and trunk to lengthen and widen? If you ask the average person to lengthen the trunk, he will raise the chest, which does not lengthen the trunk at all because it causes the back to arch and narrow; this in turn throws the rib cage backwards and causes the ribs to become fixed. In order for the trunk to truly lengthen, the back must be permitted to widen and fill out so that the ribs, which of course are in back as well as in front, can rise freely and allow breathing to take place fully and naturally (Fig. 9-7).

This same principle holds true for breathing and vocalization. Because we are more aware of the front of our bodies than the back, we are likely to assume that, in order to get air into the lungs, we must raise the chest. Actually, however, the back of the rib cage is a crucial part of the container which must expand for the lungs to take in air. When we raise the chest, this actually arches and

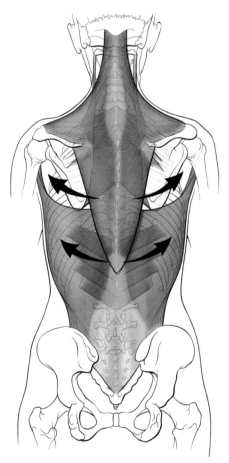

Figure 9-7. Widening of back and freeing of ribs.

narrows the back, preventing the ribs from rising and interfering with the back's natural expansion. Again, in order for the trunk truly to lengthen, the back must be able to widen and fill out, which means that the ribs in back must be able to freely expand. This allows the back to become fuller and more elastic, allowing the ribs to move easily and the trunk to support itself fully as it's designed to do (Fig. 9-7).

This expansion of the back is an integral component of the supportive network of the extensors. We saw in Chapter Two that the two deepest layers of back muscles are a key support for the upright trunk and must lengthen in order to properly fulfill their duty. But in order to fully support the trunk, the back must widen and fill out as well as lengthen. We tend to think of the muscular system in terms of maintaining postural support, which is understandable because this is one of its primary functions. But it's not enough to simply lengthen off the ground; we must do so in a way that permits flexibility and expansion in the trunk—in other words, widening. One has only to feel a narrowed back to realize that the back must be full and expansive as well as lengthened in order to properly fulfill its supportive function. When working efficiently, such an elastic, expansive back is able to support the trunk and arms without undue strain on any one part of the back because the demands placed on it are absorbed by the entire elastic network of muscular support. The back then acts as an integrated and supportive whole to maintain the support of the trunk, ribs, and shoulder girdle, and we are able to bend the trunk or use our arms to lift weight with little detectable increase in tension. When coordinated properly, the musculature is indeed a kind of suspension system, of which the lengthening and widening back is the central hub.

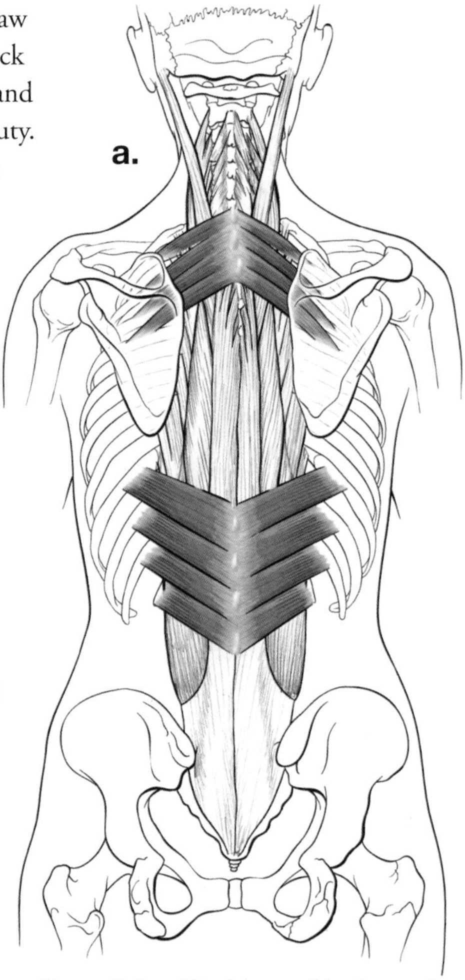

Figure 9-8a. Third layer of back muscles (serratus posterior superior and inferior).

This expansive support of the trunk involves not just the deeper layers of back muscles but the more superficial ones, which attach to the ribs and shoulder girdle. We've already seen that the two deepest layers run vertically up the back and maintain the extension of the spine and trunk; in contrast, the outer third, fourth, and fifth layers of back muscles run more horizontally and obliquely to the ribs, scapulae, and arms (Fig. 9-8). When the back lengthens, the deeper extensor muscles allow the ribs to widen; but these outer layers are also able to release in their oblique directions, which adds to the widened, elastic support of the back (Fig. 9-7).

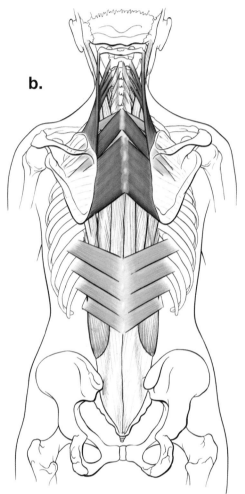

b.

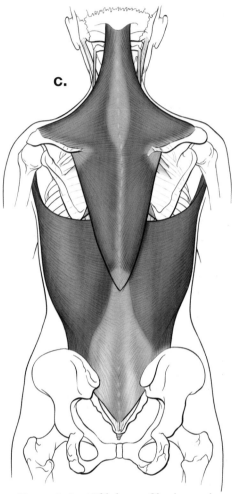

c.

Figure 9-8b. Fourth layer of back muscles (levator scapulae, rhomboid major and minor).

Figure 9-8c. Fifth layer of back muscles (trapezius and latissimus dorsi).

The proper working of the back, then, involves all five layers of back muscles, including the large "widening" muscles, such as the latissimus dorsi, and the muscles that act upon the ribs and scapulae. When this entire system is working properly, the trunk can fully discharge its supportive function through the expansive and elastic working of this multi-layered and multi-directional network of muscles.

Breathing and Our Upright Design

Although breathing is a largely automatic process, it is of course possible to improve one's breathing by deliberately drawing air into the lungs and squeezing it out, or by focusing on relaxing the belly or holding the ribs open. This has led to a common belief in the value of breathing exercises designed to increase breath flow, calm the system, and oxygenate the blood. But the benefits of such exercises are temporary and beg the question whether breathing is taking place efficiently to begin with. In fact, no breathing exercise can improve respiration if the larger system on which it depends is not working properly.

In this sense, lengthened support against gravity doesn't merely help us to breathe better. It would be more accurate to say that the elastic lengthening and widening of the back is the fundamental condition under which breathing works most efficiently; the lengthening, expansive support of the trunk is the *sine qua non* of full and efficient breathing. Like the other anatomical systems we've looked at, breathing is integrally related to, and dependent upon, our upright design. ■

10. The Voice

In the last chapter we looked at the unique role played by our upright support system in efficient breathing. As we saw, breathing is not strictly an internal process, but is intimately related to musculoskeletal function.

Let's look now at the vocal mechanism and the throat. Many books on movement and functional anatomy omit entirely any discussion of the voice, assuming that it has little relevance to movement and posture. Actually, quite the opposite is true—the voice is dependent on our upright design and in turn profoundly influences the working of the musculoskeletal system. Let's begin by looking at the larynx and how it functions to produce sound.

How We Produce Sound

The muscles of the larynx are highly specialized and somewhat complex, but when we consider the actual function of the larynx, its anatomy becomes easier to understand. Some of us learn, as children, to make a "puttering" sound by compressing our lips together and then blowing through them. Our lips begin to vibrate, creating a sound that resembles the hum of a car engine.

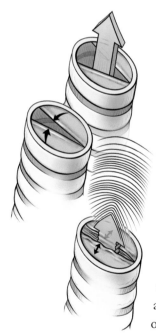

The larynx functions in much the same way as our lips when we putter. When we exhale normally, air passes unimpeded through the windpipe and out the mouth or nose. When we think of a sound, the larynx, which forms a valve at the top of the windpipe, draws the two vocal cords together; they begin to vibrate as air passes between them (Fig. 10-1). This creates sound waves which then resonate in the vocal tract—the cavities formed by the throat and mouth—to create the fully-formed tones of the human voice.

The larynx, then, is basically a vibrational mechanism. It contains oscillators that make sound (the vocal cords), and it can bring them together so that they'll vibrate when air (the power source) passes between them, and draw them back apart during normal breathing. The vocal folds themselves are also muscles and are therefore capable of tensing, which contributes to the ability of the folds to create subtle nuances in sound and expression.

Figure 10-1. When air passes between the vocal folds, they vibrate to produce sound.

Closure of the Vocal Folds

The primary function of the larynx is to open and close the vocal folds. The main housing of the larynx is the thyroid cartilage, which forms the Adam's apple on the front of the throat. The two vocal folds are situated like a "V" on the inside of the thyroid cartilage, with the pointed end of the "V" attaching to the front of the thyroid cartilage. At the other end of the "V," the vocal folds attach to two cartilages which can rotate to bring the vocal folds together and apart (Fig. 10-2). During normal breathing, the "V" is of course spread apart, so that breath passes unimpeded between the vocal folds (Fig. 10-3a). When we vocalize, however, the two rotating cartilages bring the vocal folds together (Fig. 10-3b). Air traveling between the vocal folds causes them to oscillate, which, as we've seen, creates sound.

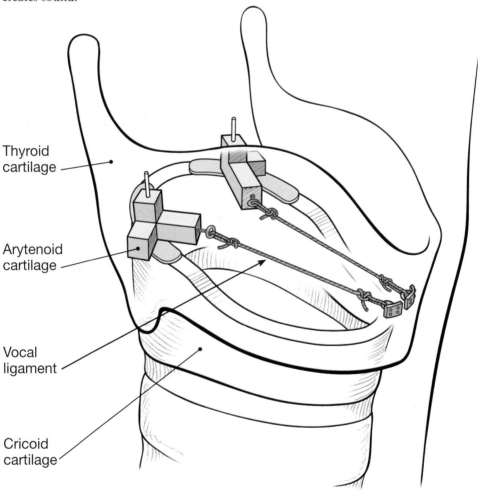

Thyroid cartilage

Arytenoid cartilage

Vocal ligament

Cricoid cartilage

Figure 10-2. Idealized depiction of the larynx, showing the two arytenoid cartilages that slide and rotate to open and close the vocal folds.

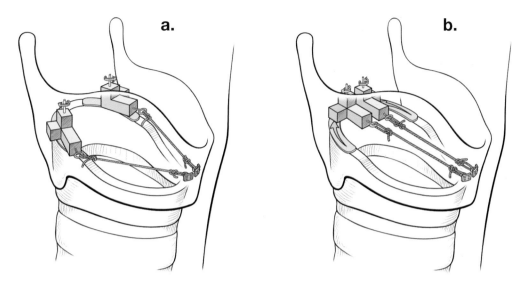

Figure 10-3. a. vocal folds open during active breathing; b. vocal folds approximated during vocalization.

It is interesting to note that, although there is one set of muscles that rotates the cartilages to open the vocal folds, the folds are actually able to close in two different ways. During normal vocalization, the vocal folds come together along their entire length and are vibrated by the flow of air, creating a normal vocalized sound (Fig. 10-3b). But the vocal folds can also close in such a way that a chink of space remains at the end where the cartilages rotate to bring them together. In this position, the vocal folds are held tightly together so that they cannot vibrate, and air coming out of the trachea escapes only through this chink, which we hear as a "whispered" sound (Fig. 10-4). Even though the vocal folds in this "whisper" position do not produced a normal vocalized sound, we can still speak, which of course makes it possible to communicate very softly.

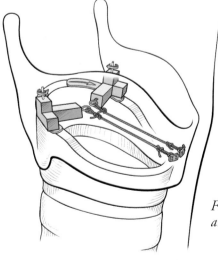

Figure 10-4. Inward rotation of arytenoid cartilages: whisper position.

The Suspensory Muscles of the Larynx

Although the larynx is a discrete organ capable of precise internal actions, it is also intimately connected with the larger musculoskeletal system. If you examine the temporal bones of the skull, which house the hearing and balancing mechanisms, you'll find two small spikes, called the styloid processes, that are set in from the sides of the skull and are therefore not visible or palpable (Fig. 10-5). Just above the larynx is a horseshoe-shaped bone, called the hyoid, which forms the base of the tongue (it is sometimes called the "tongue bone"). The larynx is suspended from this bone, which in turn is suspended from the styloid processes. The larynx is also directly suspended from the hyoid bone and anchored by muscles to the sternum below. This muscular scaffolding, sometimes called the "suspensory muscles" of the larynx, antagonistically supports the larynx from various directions (Fig. 10-6). In contrast to the muscles of the larynx itself, which form its intrinsic musculature, the suspensory muscles act upon the larynx from without and therefore constitute its extrinsic musculature.

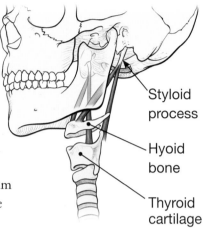

Figure 10-5. Larynx suspended from hyoid bone and styloid processes.

The suspensory muscles of the larynx play a crucial role in speaking and singing. When we hear a tenor singing a high note, for example, these muscles antagonistically pull upon the larynx from different directions to maintain the stretch on the larynx needed for it to function optimally. You can actually see changes in the position of the larynx due to the action of these muscles when you sing up a scale—in most people the larynx will visibly ascend and the throat become constricted due to the overworking of these muscles. A trained singer, on the other hand, is able to activate the suspensory muscles in such a way that the larynx is not constricted and the throat remains open; this has a marked effect on timbre, resonance, and vocal range. As we'll see in the next chapter, the ability to sing with an "open throat" depends to a large extent upon the working of the suspensory muscles of the larynx in relation to our upright posture.

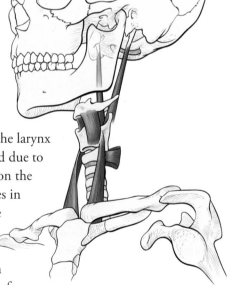

Figure 10-6. Suspensory muscles of the larynx.

The Larynx and the Breath

The working of the larynx is also intimately connected with the way we breathe. If you breathe in and out normally and then vocalize on one of the out-breaths without altering your manner of breathing, you'll notice that the resulting sound is more like a sigh than a sung tone; it will lack focus and die out very quickly—what singers call an "unsupported" tone. In contrast, a true "sung" tone has focus and clarity and can be sustained for ten seconds or more. This is because when we sing properly, the breathing and the larynx are coordinated in such a way that the breath is regulated in its flow while the vocal folds vibrate efficiently so that very little air escapes between them. When we sing and even when we speak, we aren't simply closing the vocal folds against the normal outflow of air but coordinating the two systems to produce a focused, sustained tone.

Some singers try to support the tone by tightening the abdominal muscles or expanding the ribs, which in turn increases the flow of breath through the larynx. But the vocal folds do not respond well to increased breath pressure, which creates a strained or "pressed" sound and over time can damage the vocal folds. This approach is based on the notion that, because normal exhalation is weak and "unsupported," additional muscular effort is required to produce vocal support. In reality the voice is designed in such a way that, when it's not interfered with, exhalation is naturally extended in a way that allows the vocal folds to vibrate efficiently with a minimum of air pressure. We are then able to vocalize in a seemingly effortless way, for extended periods of time.

In this sense, the larynx isn't a wind instrument and is certainly not designed to be set into motion by using brute force. When we speak or sing efficiently, the entire breathing apparatus, including our neck, trunk, back, and ribs, is automatically brought into play in a way that's finely calibrated with the closure of the vocal folds so as to create the precise amount of air flow needed to produce the intended sound. In singing, this flow must be sustained for long periods, broken up into discrete sounds, and intensified or reduced at will depending on the interpretive requirements of the music. In short, the working of the larynx requires adjustments of the subtlest sort throughout the entire musculoskeletal system, all operating in tandem to produce the full range of vocal expression.

The Larynx and the Brain

But how do the muscles of the larynx know when to bring the vocal folds together or how much to tighten? When we breathe normally, the brain automatically tells the vocal folds to stay apart, ensuring the free flow of oxygen to the lungs. However, when we want to communicate musically, as we do when we sing, the brain translates this intention into signals to the larynx which tell the vocal folds to come together while simultaneously coordinating various muscles to produce the intended sounds.

The muscles of the larynx, then, are not controlled consciously the way we control the finger muscles or even the muscles of the palate; they are controlled indirectly by the part of the brain that hears sounds, as well as by centers that produce thoughts and form words. This is why people who are born deaf are never able to acquire full control over the vocal muscles: with no experience of sound, they are unable to fully engage the centers of the brain that control the muscles involved in the formation of speech and song.

The larynx thus exhibits a range and precision of action that is unparalleled anywhere else in the body. By coordinating the muscles of breathing with the closure of the larynx, the vibratory mechanism of the larynx is brought into play in the most exquisite and subtle manner. By controlling the delicate musculature of the vocal folds, we control the pitch and create different sound textures. By activating the muscular scaffolding of the throat, the larynx is suspended antagonistically within its muscular network with the exact amount of tension required for the athletic act of hitting a high "C" or singing over a full orchestra. And functioning as both composer and conductor, the brain orchestrates all of this activity to produce the glorious and expressive sounds of the human voice—a true marvel of engineering and design. ∎

11. The Suspensory Muscles of the Throat

In the last chapter we saw that the larynx, which forms a valve at the top of the windpipe, consists of two vocal fold muscles that are suspended within the thyroid cartilage and the two arytenoid cartilages, which by rotating can bring the vocal folds together or draw them apart. When we breathe normally, the vocal folds are drawn apart so that air can pass freely between them. When the vocal folds are brought together, air passing between them causes them to vibrate, which creates sound waves that resonate in the cavities above.

As we've also seen, the larynx, marvelous and complex as it is in its own right, is not an isolated and discrete organ. Because it evolved in conjunction with breathing, the larynx works cooperatively with the respiratory system to produce sound. It is also supported by a network of muscles which pull upon it from different directions to assist the stretching of the vocal folds in creating particular pitches and qualities of sound. Let's look now at this throat musculature and its relation to our upright support system.

The Suspended Throat

If you look at an anatomical drawing of the front of the neck, you'll see that the muscles in this region form an intricate network or webbing at the throat and the underside of the jaw (Fig. 11-1). The function of these muscles, in addition to vocalization and speech, is to assist in such basic life functions as eating, breathing, and swallowing. Though this region is far and away the most complex part of the human musculature and includes dozens of muscles, it is usually omitted from books on the anatomy of movement, no doubt because it has little involvement in overt action.

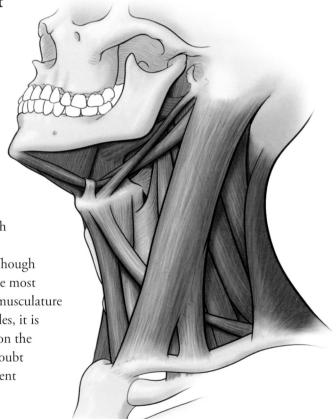

Figure 11-1. The network of throat muscles.

These muscles, however, are integral to our upright support system and profoundly influence the working of the musculo-skeletal system as a whole. We saw in the last chapter that the hyoid bone and larynx are suspended from the styloid processes at the base of the skull (Fig. 11-2). The muscles of the throat, or pharynx, are also hung from the skull just in front of the foramen magnum, the hole in the base of the skull through which the spinal cord extends down the spine (Fig. 11-3). And the jaw, which articulates with the temporal bone to form the temporo-mandibular joint, is slung from this joint and from muscles attaching to the sides of the skull (Fig. 11-4). In other words, all the main structures of the throat hang from the skull and, as we shall see, are closely involved in the workings of the upright support system.

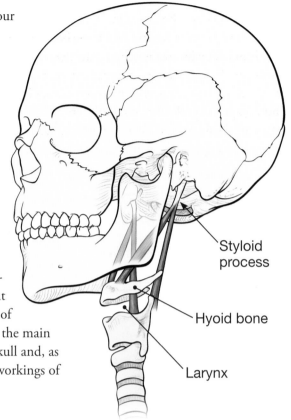

Styloid process

Hyoid bone

Larynx

Figure 11-2. Hyoid bone and larynx suspended from styloid processes.

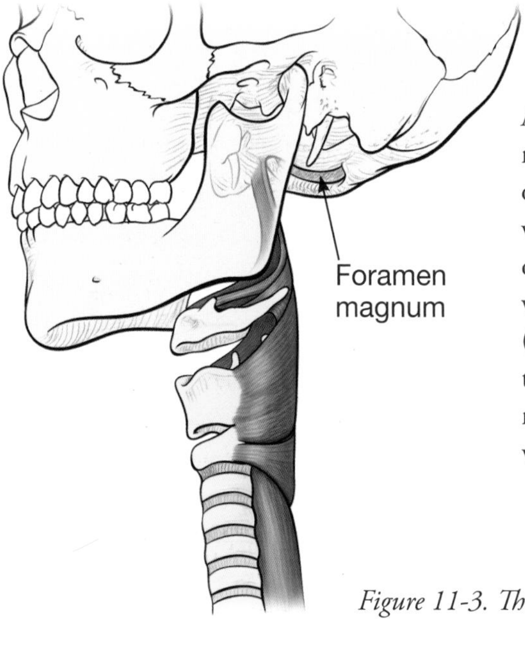

Foramen magnum

As we saw in the last chapter, the musculature of the throat is a crucial part of the singing and speaking apparatus. When we sing, these muscles antagonistically pull on the larynx from different directions, which is needed for it to function optimally (Fig. 11-5). A singer must be able to activate these suspensory muscles, which has a marked effect on timbre, resonance, and vocal range.

Figure 11-3. Throat suspended from base of skull.

This musculature also assists in supporting the upper spinal column and in counteracting the pull of the extensor muscles at the back of the neck. In four-footed animals, the head tends to fall by its own weight, so the flexors on the underside of the neck are relatively weak and few in number. In upright humans, the rather weak neck flexors can easily be overpowered by the powerful backward pull of the neck extensors. To prevent this from happening, the throat muscles are called into play to assist the neck flexors; this can clearly be seen in wrestlers and track-and-field athletes whose throat muscles bulge when they're performing strenuous movements.

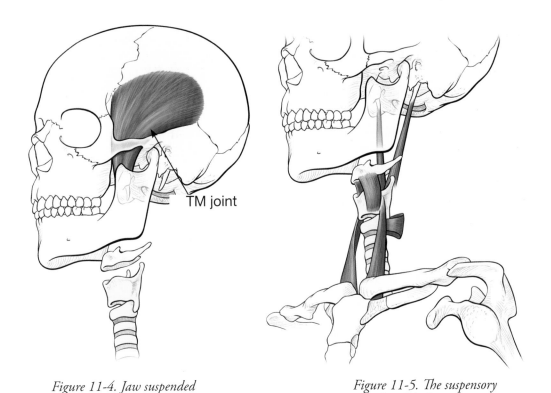

Figure 11-4. Jaw suspended from temporal bones.

Figure 11-5. The suspensory muscles of the larynx.

Depressing the Larynx

But the muscles of the throat are not mainly postural in function, and this is where the problem comes in. In order to function properly, the larynx, tongue, and jaw must hang freely from the skull without upsetting the balance of the head on the spine. When we are able to maintain the length and support of this larger system, the throat remains open and the muscles that act upon the larynx can work freely. In tenors with pillar-like necks, for example, the neck and throat muscles are naturally well-developed and provide a stable support for the larynx. The throat is open and free, and the larynx can be actively engaged during the athletic activity of singing without any sense of effort or strain.

Over time, however, many of us use the voice in such a way that we collapse and tighten the throat. The musculature of the throat becomes constricted and the larynx is pulled downward by the tugging of muscles that are overworked. This creates a drag on the skull and the upper spinal column and compromises the length of the trunk, thus interfering with the upright support system (Fig. 11-6).

A number of factors contribute to the tightening of the throat muscles, but perhaps the main one is harmful habits of speech. People who use the voice in a heavy, enervated manner tend to collapse the musculature of the throat, resulting in a hoarse, throaty tone of voice; prolonged speaking in this way can have a depressive and devitalizing effect on the entire system. Professional speakers and singers often develop harmful patterns of tension in the muscles of the neck and ribs, habitually tensing the throat muscles and gasping for air between phrases.

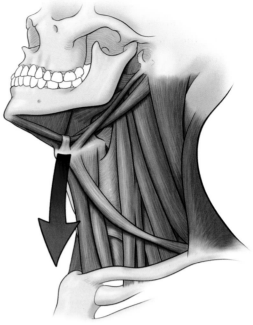

Figure 11-6. Throat muscles dragging on the skull.

A sedentary lifestyle can also contribute to the tendency to collapse the palate, tongue, and throat. While working at a desk, many people collapse the palate and, instead of breathing freely through the nostrils, breathe heavily through the mouth. Even while sleeping, many of us collapse and tighten the throat muscles in such a way that they drag upon the head and spine.

The Throat and Upright Poise

The flexors of the throat, then, constitute a key system that must be taken into account if we are to fully understand our upright design. In Chapter Three we saw that the rib cage and innards tend to pull down in the front of the body, contributing to the tendency to lose length. As we've just seen, the structures of the throat can also pull down in front, dragging upon the head and the upper spinal column. As long as the throat is constricted in this way, the head cannot balance freely upon the spine, and the upper spinal column and trunk cannot fully lengthen. The suspensory muscles of the throat, in this case, contribute to the overall tendency to interfere with our upright support. Conversely, a freely suspended throat that does not drag on the skull is an essential component of our ability to lengthen against gravity.

Notice also the effect this "flexor sheet" has on the balance of the head. As we saw earlier, the extensor muscles attached to the back of the skull tend to pull the head back, while the forward weight of the head on the spine counterbalances this tendency. The same is true of the flexors in front: their attachments to the mastoid processes are slightly behind the point of balance of the skull and therefore they also pull the head back. The styloid processes, on the other hand, are slightly in *front* of the point of balance of the skull (Fig. 11-7—see red arrows). This means that the throat muscles, instead of pulling the head back and down, actually pull it down and forward, just as one would expect (Fig. 11-8a).

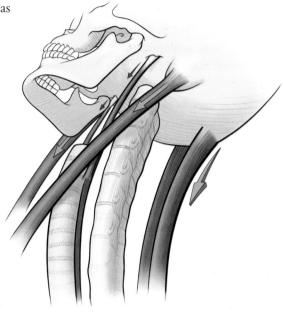

Figure 11-7. The styloid processes are in front of the point of balance of the skull.

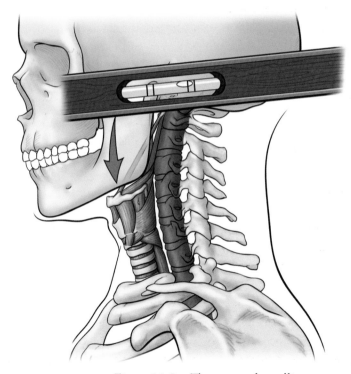

Figure 11-8a. Throat muscles pulling the skull down and forward.

When the throat musculature is not unduly contracted, however, the downward drag on the skull is eased and the structures of the throat, including the larynx within its muscular scaffolding, become properly suspended from above (Fig. 11-8b). This results in a freer, more open use of the voice while at the same time allowing the body to regain its optimal length.

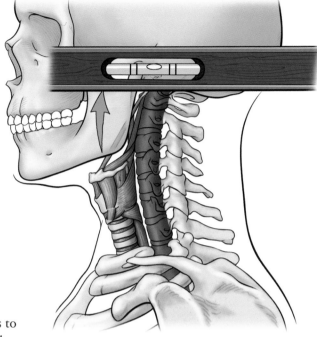

The "Open Throat"

This relation of the throat muscles to our upright posture is the key to the desirable condition sought by singers known as an "open throat." We've seen

Figure 11-8b. Free suspension of throat muscles: an open throat.

that the jaw, larynx, and throat are all suspended from the skull. If we shorten and collapse this musculature, the muscular webbing of the larynx and throat and underside of the jaw tightens and the throat itself becomes collapsed and closed. Since the throat is flexible and largely formed by the surrounding musculature, it is profoundly affected by the degree of tightness of this musculature, which in turn affects vocal quality.

When, on the other hand, the head goes up as it is designed to do, this network of throat muscles also releases. The larynx, which as we've seen hangs from its suspensory muscles and is stretched antagonistically during the act of vocalizing, is now able to function optimally. The tongue and throat, freely suspended from the skull, no longer impinge upon the larynx, and the pharynx becomes mobile and open (Fig. 11-8b).

There are many methods that seek to open the throat by altering the shape of the pharynx, raising the soft palate, and "placing" the voice during singing. But while partially effective, these techniques are not based on a complete understanding of the design of the throat musculature and its ultimate dependence on head balance and upright poise. Truly open-throated singing occurs naturally when the overall support system hasn't been interfered with and the throat musculature is freely suspended from the skull. We can hear what an open throat sounds like in the clear, piercing, and uninhibited voices of young children. To an almost universal extent, they haven't yet learned to interfere with the upright support system, which holds the key to the release of the suspensory muscles of larynx.

The Jaw

The same principle applies to the jaw. The function of the jaw is to chew and grind food, and for this purpose it's hinged with and hung from the skull at the temporomandibular or TM joint (the joint formed by the temporal bone of the skull and the mandible) and acted upon by three sets of powerful muscles which often become chronically tense, limiting the freedom and mobility of the jaw. It's easy to assume that this tension can be alleviated by moving the jaw or attempting to relax these muscles directly. As we've seen, however, the jaw is inseparably linked with the structures on the underside of the jaw, including the tongue, hyoid bone, and larynx; any tension in this area pulls on the jaw and causes the jaw muscles to compensate by tightening (Fig. 11-9). For this reason, exercises for freeing the jaw muscles fail to address the underlying cause of tension in the jaw. In contrast, when the muscles of the throat are able to release so that the head is balanced forward on the skull and the throat muscles, instead of pulling on the skull, are freely suspended from the skull, the jaw muscles release sympathetically. Again, the balanced working of the larger support system holds the key to the freedom of the jaw.

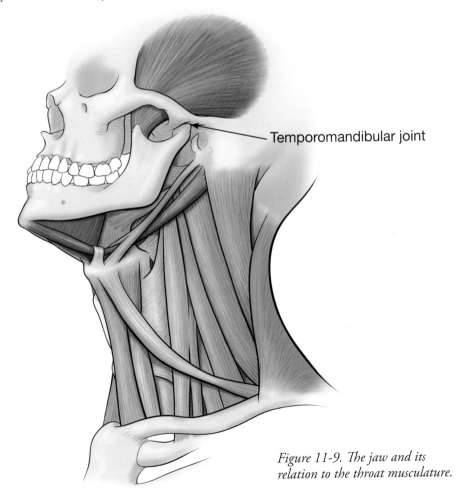

Temporomandibular joint

Figure 11-9. The jaw and its relation to the throat musculature.

Head Balance Revised

To recap, there are three key groups of muscles attaching to the base of the skull. The two largest systems are the extensors running along the back of the body and the flexors in front. The extensors attach at the back of the skull and therefore pull the head back. The flexors in front attach via the sternomastoid muscle to the mastoid process of the skull and also pull the head back (Fig. 11-10a). As we've seen, these two systems support the trunk against gravity so that we are able to stand upright.

The third and final system is the musculature of the throat and larynx, which is suspended from the base of the skull and forms part of the system of flexors on the front of the neck.

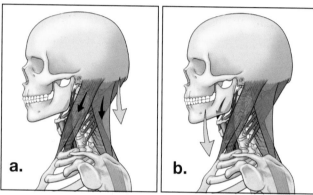

Figure 11-10. The three muscle systems attaching to the base of the skull.

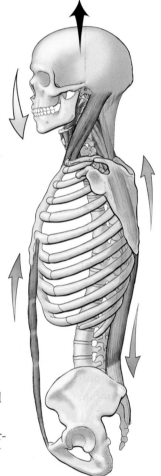

Like the rib cage and abdomen below it, the throat contributes to the tendency to pull down and collapse in front. Unlike the larger flexor sheet, however, the throat muscles attach slightly in front of the point of balance of the skull; if we misuse the throat or voice, these muscles can exert excessive drag on the head, causing it to be pulled forward and down (Fig. 11-10b). We saw earlier that the head must freely tilt forward in such a way that it activates the extensors of the back while not interfering with lengthening in the front—that is, it must go forward and up, not forward and down. Because the suspensory muscles of the throat tend to pull down on the skull, it's especially important that the skull move upward in order to ensure the release of this crucial muscular network (Fig. 11-11). Only then can the throat "let go" of the head, allowing the spine to regain its full length as the head releases upward. In this sense, the voice is a crucial part of the muscular system and can influence it in profound ways, which is why any system of movement is incomplete that does not take into account the jaw, tongue, and the suspensory muscles of the voice and throat. ■

Figure 11-11. The three muscle systems in relation to head balance.

12. The Spiral Musculature

In the last chapter we looked at the musculature of the throat. Along with the extensors on the back of the body and the flexors in front, it forms a third system that attaches to the skull and is intimately involved in upright support. Let's look now at the oblique or spiral muscles that wrap around the trunk and limbs, and the special role they play in our upright design.

Rotational Movement and Our Upright Design

In earlier chapters we saw that there's a large extensor sheet running up the length of the back from the sacrum to the base of the skull. We also saw that counterbalancing this extensor sheet is the flexor sheet on the front of the body which we traced from the pubic bone to the rib cage and from there to the mastoid process of the skull. However, this description is over-simplified. A quick glance at a muscle chart reveals that most of the muscles of the trunk run at oblique angles, diagonally encircling the abdomen and ribs (Fig. 12-1). This is also true, though to a lesser extent, of the extensor muscles in back, many of which do not run vertically but also slant at oblique angles.

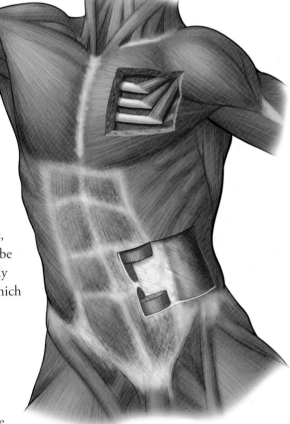

The reason for this design feature is that, in order to move efficiently, we need to be able not only to flex and extend the body but to rotate it. In primitive animals, which lack oblique muscles, a crude rotation is accomplished by the asymmetrical contraction of one segment of the body in relation to another. Later vertebrates developed oblique or slanting muscles that wrap around the trunk and limbs and could therefore produce much more efficient torquing or twisting movements

Figure 12-1. Oblique muscles of the trunk.

of the body; this can be observed very strikingly in cats when they fall upside down and right themselves in mid-air, twisting their bodies and landing on their feet.

No vertebrate, however, is capable of twisting movements as complex as those of humans, whose two-footed upright posture makes it possible to twist or gyrate the trunk around a vertical axis, and to rotate the head independently of the body (Fig. 12-2). Our ability to use tools, to play musical instruments, to write and draw—in short, many of our most prized skills—are based on our unique ability to twist or rotate our bodies.

The Evolution of Spiral Muscles

Let's explore for a moment how the spiral muscles evolved. In fish, as we've seen, muscles are arranged segmentally along either side of the body so that the body can be flexed from side to side to produce forward movement in the water. The musculature is also divided into the dorsal and ventral parts—that is, the extensors on the back side of the fish and the flexors on the belly side (Fig. 12-3). A fish can only flex its body from side to side, but in various species these two muscle divisions—those on either side of the body and those on the front and back—produce two kinds of movement: lateral flexion, and extension and flexion. In species such as worms, these two types of movement can be combined to produce a primitive form of twisting.

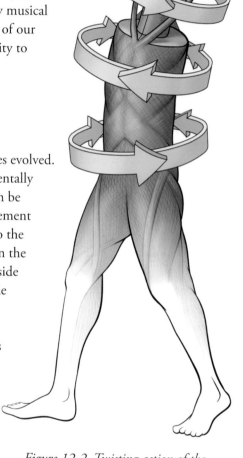

Figure 12-2. Twisting action of the trunk with the head rotating on top.

Vertebrates that came onto land developed a much more sophisticated musculature in response to the need to expand the range of motor abilities. We've seen that amphibians and reptiles used their limbs as levers to raise themselves off the ground; the spine became, in essence, a bridge supporting the internal organs and ribs which hung below. The extensor muscles in back now supported the spine and helped to maintain extension of the limbs; the flexor muscles wrapped around the entire abdominal region and rib cage. In order to efficiently rotate or twist the trunk, flexor muscles that wrapped around the trunk in a slanting or oblique direction were needed. This presented a problem, however, since there were no muscles running in oblique directions, and because the established bilateral

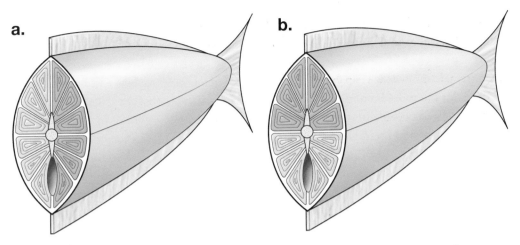

Figure 12-3. The two basic muscle divisions: a. lateral; b. dorsal and ventral.

body plan prevented muscles from crossing the midline to form a continuous sheet of muscles wrapping around the trunk.

To solve the problem, the flexor muscles on the trunk divided into three layers. The deepest layer ran horizontally, but the middle and superficial layers took a different course and developed in oblique directions. Two layers of abdominal and thoracic muscles now wrapped around the trunk at oblique angles, combining with the rotational muscles of the neck and spine to allow the complex twisting movements so essential to efficient movement on land (Fig. 12-4).

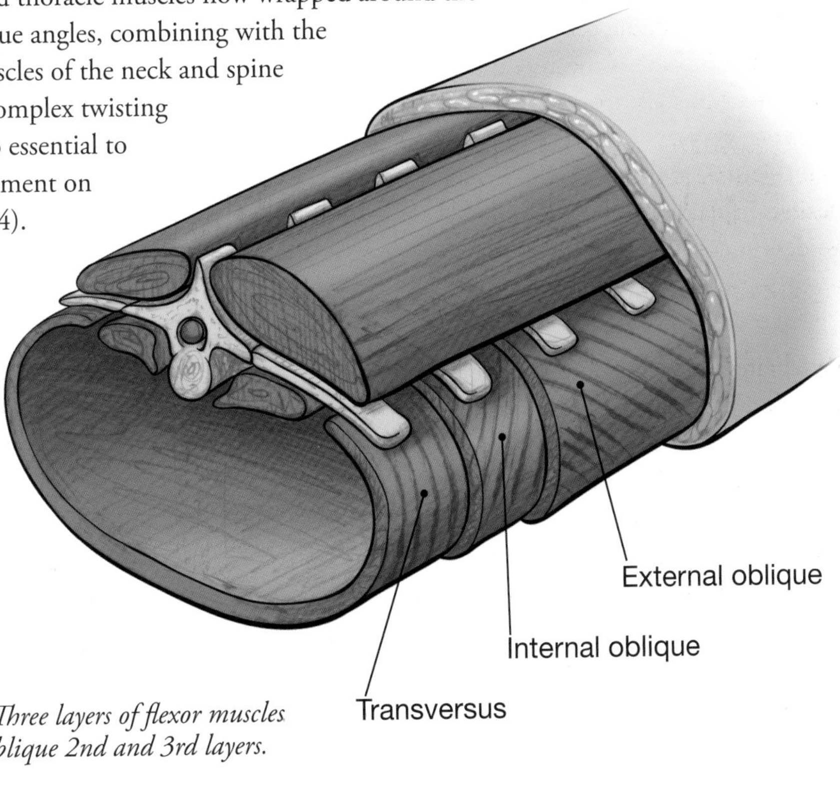

External oblique

Internal oblique

Transversus

Figure 12-4. Three layers of flexor muscles showing the oblique 2nd and 3rd layers.

In humans, these oblique muscles have evolved to permit an even more efficient rotation around a vertical axis (see Fig. 12-2). This advanced design, however, is built upon the foundation of the basic body plan established eons ago in our vertebrate ancestors. In keeping with our bilateral design, the muscles that wrap around our ribs and abdomen do not cross the abdominal midline. There are also no muscles that cross from one side of the back to the other. But when you piece together a complete pattern by identifying an oblique muscle in one layer and then find another muscle layer on the other side of the midline that continues in the same direction, it's possible to trace a continuous spiral that begins at the pelvis, wraps around the trunk, and ends up at the base of the skull (Fig. 12-5). And we can do this in both directions, so that we can trace two complete spirals running from the pelvis right up to the head, one on each side, forming a complex double-spiral that encircles the body and continues even into the limbs, making complex rotational movements possible.

Rotational Movement and the Use of the Arms

As I said, this spiral musculature is central to our ability, as humans, to perform many of our most complex activities. In Chapter Five we saw how the movable shoulder girdle contributes to the range of motion of the arm. If you perform a throwing or swinging action, you can see that it is also necessary, when moving the arm, to rotate the trunk and even the legs. In other words, the use of the arm and shoulder is continuous with the twisting and spiraling action of the entire body. Observe a track and field athlete throwing a javelin, a violinist vigorously bowing, or even an artist drawing at an easel and it's easy to see that these complex uses of the arms—indeed, many of our most refined abilities as humans—require the ability to rotate the trunk. When viewed in terms of the spiral musculature, in fact, it is clear that few movements occur in two planes; virtually all movement takes place in three dimensions, including the spiral or rotational movement of the trunk.

Anatomy of the Spiral Musculature

Let's now trace one of these muscular spirals in the trunk, beginning at the right side of the pelvis in front. The internal oblique muscle on the right side of the abdomen originates at the anterior rim of the pelvis and runs obliquely upward to the midline of the abdomen, or linea alba (Fig. 12-5a). If you cross the midline and continue in the same direction, you'll be following the external oblique abdominis muscle on the left side as it runs obliquely upward and out (Fig. 12-5b). The line is continued by the external intercostal muscle which wraps around the rib cage to the upper back on the left side, intersects with the levatores costarum and the transverse processes of the cervical vertebrae, and again crosses the midline of the spine (Fig. 12-5c). The line is then continued by the right splenius capitis muscle, which originates at the transverse processes on the right side of upper spine and runs upward to attach finally to the right occiput (Fig. 12-5d).

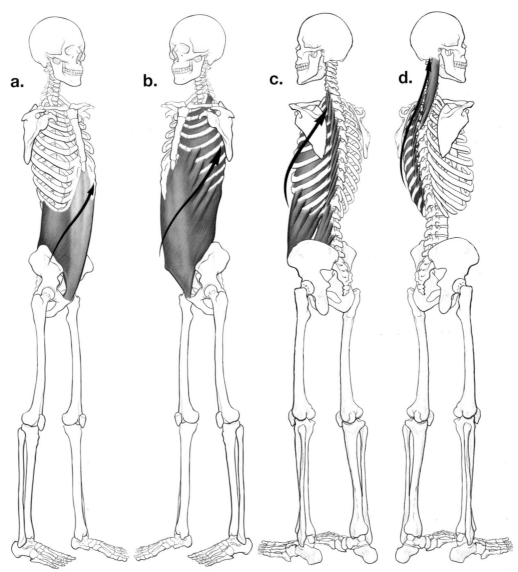

Figure 12-5. One of the key spirals wrapping around the trunk from pelvis to occiput.

So, beginning from the pelvis, it is possible to trace a continuous spiral of muscle pulls that begins at the right anterior rim of the pelvis, crosses the abdomen to the rib cage on the left side, circles around the ribs to the back, continues obliquely across the transverse processes of the cervical vertebrae in back, and finally ends at the occiput on the same side as it began.

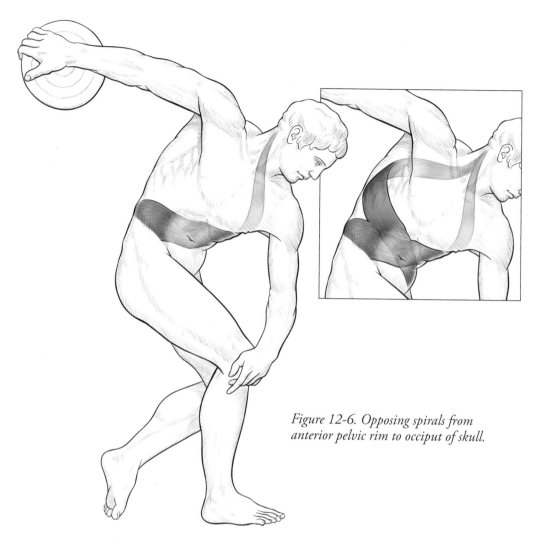

Figure 12-6. Opposing spirals from anterior pelvic rim to occiput of skull.

An identical spiral can be traced on the opposite side, so that we end up with two interlacing spirals wrapping around the trunk (Fig. 12-6).

We can also trace each of the two spirals from different starting points. If, for example, you begin the first spiral, not at the anterior right rim of the pelvis, but at the back of the pelvis on the left side, the spiral now crosses the midline in back, wraps around the right side of the rib cage to the right side of the sternum, crosses the midline, and continues from the origin of the left sternocleidomastoid muscle at the top of the sternum to its attachment at the left mastoid process. Another spiral can be traced from the right posterior rim of the pelvis to the right mastoid process (Fig. 12-7). Thus the musculature of the trunk can be viewed, not simply as a series of muscles that support us in our upright posture, but as a system of spiral muscles that can twist or torque the body in different ways.

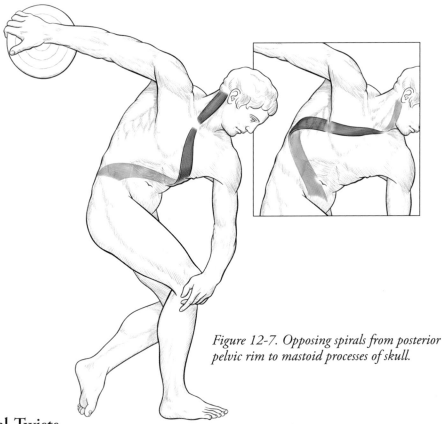

Figure 12-7. Opposing spirals from posterior pelvic rim to mastoid processes of skull.

Postural Twists

Although our bodies are designed to rotate, when we perform skilled work with tools or other instruments in which one hand is dominant, constant rotation or torquing can cause our musculature to become habitually twisted. We can observe such postural twisting in a child learning to write or a programmer working in front of a computer; it constitutes one of the major causes of shortening and collapsing the muscular system. Some degree of spinal twisting, in fact, is present in virtually all of us, particularly if we are engaged in skilled work which involves dominance on one side and therefore a constant asymmetrical twisting of the body.

Restoring optimal function requires an untwisting and freeing of the neck and trunk, which allows the body to become symmetrical and properly released into its full length. Since the spiral muscles that wrap around the trunk ultimately attach to the head, postural twists always involve a pulling back of the head, which is why the balance of the head is as crucial to maintaining the natural length of the spiral musculature as it was to maintaining the length of the extensor muscles running lengthwise down the back. When this system is working properly, the head balances forward so that the trunk can untwist and lengthen. In this sense, the spiral musculature doesn't so much pull on the head as hang suspended from it; ultimately, the head leads and the body is suspended from the head.

The Suspended Trunk: Our Fishy Ancestry

But what does it mean to say that the body is suspended from the head by means of these spirals, and why is the relationship of the head to the trunk the main organizing principle governing the spiral musculature? We've seen that early vertebrates moved toward food by levering the spine laterally with the aid of muscles arranged along each side of the body. The body of the fish literally swings from the head to produce the lateral undulations of swimming (Fig. 12-8).

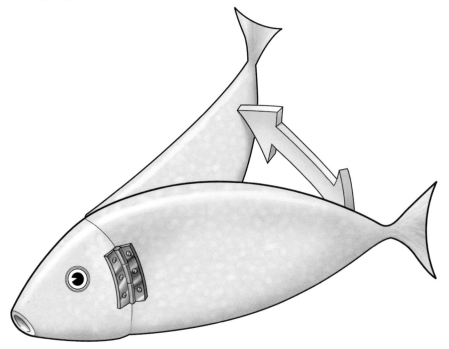

Figure 12-8. Fish with the body swinging from the head.

Animals that came onto land needed to support themselves up off the ground in order to use their limbs for locomotion. The spine then becomes a horizontal bridge with the head extending out from the body. Extensor muscles on the neck support the head while extensors on the back support the body on extended limbs. Amphibians and reptiles flex the body sideways to advance their limbs; mammals are able to coil and extend their bodies to push off with their legs. But the relationship of the head to the body organizes movement regardless, and even in mammals the body essentially swings from the head, as we can see when a dog wags its tail and the tail wags the body, or when it runs (Fig. 12-9).

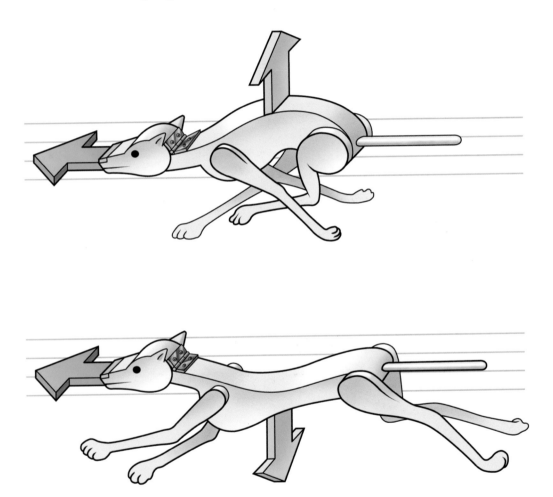

Figure 12-9. Four-footed animal with the extensor muscles countered by the forward weight of the head, but with the body still swinging from the head.

In primates and particularly in humans, this arrangement is altered yet again. The spine is up-ended, and the head, which no longer hangs out in front of the spine but now sits up on top of it, is delicately poised off-center on the spine to counter the backward pull of the extensor muscles. The body is still hung, or suspended, from the skull, just as it is in a fish or four-footed animal, and the relationship of the head to the trunk remains the primary factor organizing the upright support system (Fig. 12-10a).

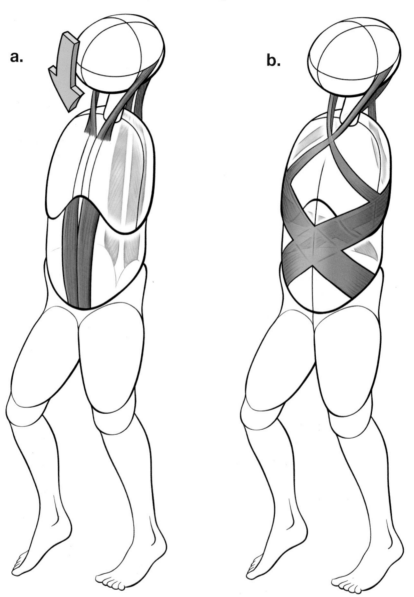

Figure 12-10. Human design: a. head conterpoised on top of the spine to maintain the length of the trunk, and the body swinging from the head; b. head conterpoised on top of the spine, but with the body swinging from the head in the form of two spirals.

But one other crucial change occurred in the process of attaining upright posture. Because the body is vertically poised on a narrow base of two feet with the head balanced on top of the spine, the oblique muscles that wrap around the neck, trunk, and limbs make it possible to rotate the body very efficiently around a vertical axis—an all-important development because it granted human beings a 360-degree field of vision, the ability to walk with a striding gait, and the possibility of mastering a huge array of skilled activities. The lateral flexion of lizards and dogs is long gone. We are still hung from the head; the relationship of the head to the trunk is still the primary relationship organizing movement; but we are hung, not just side to side as in a fish or front to back as in a mammal, but in a double spiral that permits the performance of complex rotational movements (Fig. 12-10b). We need only to watch a dancer executing a perfect pirouette, a golfer swinging a club, or a martial artist gyrating in the air to land a well-placed kick on an opponent to understand that, in movement, the body swings from the head. We are not merely stacked up or aligned over our feet; we are actually suspended from the skull, with the musculature of the trunk and the legs arranged underneath in a double-spiral—an altogether extraordinary structure.

Our Double-Helix Architecture

We have all observed the beautiful and elegant spiral designs that seem to abound in the universe—spiral nebulae, climbing vines, an elephant's trunk, the coiled musculature of the human heart and intestines—and of course the structure of DNA, with its famous double-helix arrangement containing our genetic blueprint. It is fascinating to consider that our evolution to a fully upright posture recapitulates in our musculo-skeletal system the same elegant spiral design that's embedded at a microscopic level in our own DNA—a design largely responsible for our varied and complex capabilities as humans. We may be one of many evolutionary "experiments," but our upright design is the most highly refined and sophisticated in the known universe. And whereas the double-helix structure of DNA is comprised of two spirals turning in the same direction (like the two rails of a spiral staircase), our musculature consists of two interlocking spirals, each of which is a kind of double-helix in its own right—a *double* double-helix! (Fig. 12-11)

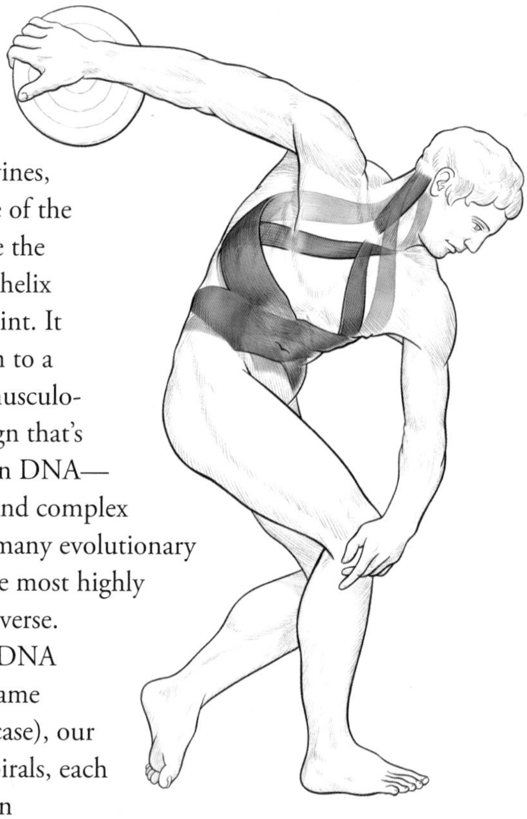

Figure 12-11. Double spiral musculature.

Lengthening into the Spirals

We've seen that the flexors on the front of the body and the extensors in back form crucial systems that maintain upright support, and that both of these systems attach to the head, whose forward balance counteracts the downward pull of these muscles. The same principle applies to the spiral muscles that wrap around the body, which also attach to the head and are counterbalanced by its forward tilt on the spine. When this system works as it is designed to work, the shoulders float lightly above the rib cage, the throat is freely suspended from the skull, the back is full and supportive, and the entire structure rotates freely on a vertical axis, making for the elegant and complex human design that expresses such variety of action, subtlety of movement, and beauty of form. ■

13. The Miracle of the Human Form

For all its complexity, the human body exhibits a remarkable logic and elegance in its design. The spine, the shoulder girdle, the voice, the pelvis and legs—each part is beautifully suited for its particular function. Central to these systems is our upright posture—the vertical balance of our trunk on our legs that makes it possible for us to stride easily on two feet, to move in an infinite variety of ways, to manipulate objects with our hands and arms, to form speech, and to perform the complex rotational movements that underlie many of our most sophisticated skills.

Our Upright Suspension System

As we've seen, we are able to stand upright not simply because our bones are stacked one on top of the other, or because muscles pull on parts of the body like guy wires to keep us from falling over. The body is a dynamic suspension system that enables muscles to support from above as well as to act from below. When our upright support system works in accordance with its design, the effect is to produce upward support with a minimum of effort—a paradoxical dynamic much like that of a tent being supported by guy wires. At the same time that the guy wires "tighten" to keep the tent pole from falling, the pole itself actually stretches the guy wires. In much the same way, the human form, when properly poised, seems to spring upward effortlessly against gravity, maintaining its vertical thrust because muscles supporting the head and trunk from below are also being lengthened from above.

This dynamic support system is the crucial foundation for the skilled activities that characterize us as a species. We must learn, as children, to throw a ball, to balance on skates, or to play the violin. But we are able to master such complex skills only because our system is perfectly designed to permit a wide array of movements while maintaining fluid balance on two feet. The cortex plays a crucial role in learning, but our broad repertoire of human abilities—the dexterous use of the arm and hand, the ability to move and to produce sound with our voices, athletic and dance movements—are entirely dependent on our upright support system and its subtle and remarkable design.

Our upright support system also holds the key to the proper functioning of specific systems. Specific exercises for aligning and strengthening parts of the body such as the lower back may produce immediate benefits in functioning. But as we've seen, the muscles of the lower back are inextricably linked with the larger upright system and can function properly only in this context. The same holds true for the balanced working of the body as a whole. Exercises for improving alignment, for relaxing and toning muscles, or for improving breathing often produce a sense of increased well-being. But unless we understand the body's total design, we are skirting around the edges of a more fundamental problem. The body is designed as a total system to support itself against gravity and, when this system is working well, to move and function with fluid grace. Understanding how this system works is the most important knowledge we can possess about the health and functioning of the musculoskeletal system.

Our Unique Design Features

We are accustomed, as humans, to feel that we have risen above our biological heritage, and to value most highly those cognitive and intellectual attributes that we view as independent of, or superior to, our physical nature. But our humanity expresses itself as much in our physical design as in our higher-order mental faculties. Our speech, our striding gait, our ability to sit at a piano or at the dinner table, our gestures and manners—these physical attributes are as much a part of our humanity as our higher mental functions.

Even our cognitive abilities, which seem to emanate directly from our brains, are intimately related to our physical design. As we saw earlier in this book, four-footed animals such as wolves and rabbits are able to think and to process information, but always in the service of immediate physical action. This link between thought and action is reflected in their horizontal physical design: sensory information processed at the front end, or head, is translated directly into forward movement in space. In contrast, we humans are no longer "locked in" to movement but are designed to look at what is around us, to stop and think. In coming to the fully upright posture, humans have developed the capacity to separate thought and action, to defer immediate response and to work toward ends often far removed from the initial stimuli which set them into motion. This uniquely human capacity for autonomy and choice is directly related to our upright design.

It is no coincidence that our most sophisticated activities are all conducted in the upright posture. We perform mental calculations, write, draw, use tools and play musical instruments, meditate, and speak while fully upright (often sitting so that we are even further removed from physical activity), and only assume a horizontal position when we are unconscious and need to rest. Even athletic and physical skills, which are often performed in a crouching position, ultimately gain benefit from the fully upright position: the greatest martial arts masters and other high-level performers often achieve total mastery only after undergoing long periods of meditation in a balanced, quiet state of vertical poise. In short, none of our higher functions exists independently of our physical design, without which we would be incapable of creative thinking, invention, spirituality, technology, and the arts, and without which the human brain itself could not have evolved.

Our upright poise is also connected with our spiritual qualities, which are reflected in our ability to stand in awe of the world around us and to contemplate the universe. Like all living things, we are rooted in biological processes, but we humans alone among the animals possess the dual qualities of being grounded in the earth while reaching ever upward. In the act of becoming fully upright, we have become spiritually dignified.

Our Higher-Order Design

The human organism is the most complex piece of machinery on the planet, a thing so vast that it is a world unto itself. We recognize in the autonomy and uniqueness of each individual, and in the individual course each of us sets in life, a purposefulness that transcends our animal natures. But something about each component in our physical design leads to purpose: the use of the upper limb, which makes it possible to build, invent, create art, and explore the world; the use of the voice, which makes expression and communication possible; our highly developed senses and mental faculties; our fully upright, poised balance, which imbues life with a contemplative, spiritual dimension. None of our distinctive human attributes would exist without this design; it invests us with our sense of beauty and is the instrument by means of which our greatest intellectual, moral, technological, artistic, and spiritual achievements are made possible.

The human body is a true miracle of nature, with which we are each endowed at birth. We should celebrate this physical form, so imbued with mind and spirit, and sing praise to its beauty. ■

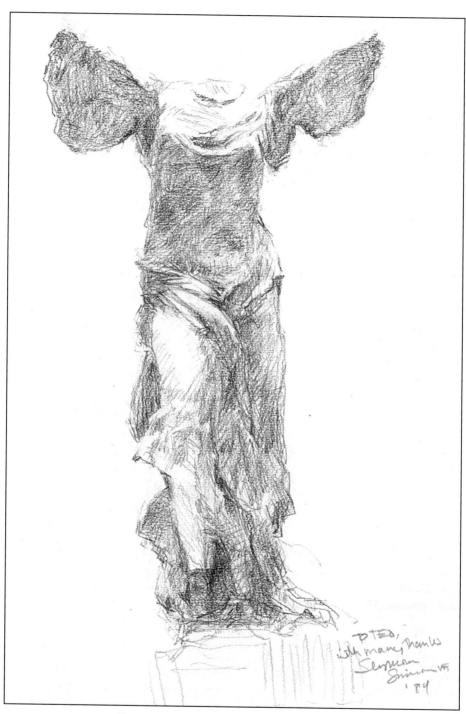

Figure 13-1. Winged Victory of Samothrace.

Index

About the Author

The director of the Dimon Institute in New York City, Theodore Dimon, Jr., EdD, teaches and lectures internationally. He became certified to teach the Alexander Technique in 1983 at the Constructive Teaching Centre in London, England, and is a founding director of the American Society for the Alexander Technique. He received both master's and doctorate degrees in education from Harvard University. Dimon has developed an innovative theory of education that focuses on mastery of mind and body as the foundation for all learning. He is the author of *Anatomy of the Moving Body*, Second Edition; *The Elements of Skill*; *The Undivided Self*; and *Your Body, Your Voice*.

About the Illustrator

A medical illustrator with twenty-six years of experience, G. David Brown earned his undergraduate degree from Harvard University and his master's degree in medical illustration from the University of Texas Health Science Center at Dallas. In his current position, Brown runs the bachelor of fine arts illustration program at Winthrop University in Rock Hill, South Carolina, where he trains young illustrators in the art and science of medical illustration.